Cardiovascular Wellness Management Success Plan

A SIMPLE, COST EFFECTIVE 3-STEP SYSTEM TO DIAGNOSE, TREAT, MONITOR AND ERADICATE HEART ATTACKS AND STROKES FROM YOUR PRACTICE WHILE GROWING YOUR BOTTOM LINE

BY TODD C. ELDREDGE PhD

Healthy Heart Publishing

9677 South 700 East, Sandy UT. 84020

www.healthyheartco.com

vs 1.5

Cardiovascular Wellness Management Success Plan

A Simple, Cost Effective, 3-Step System to Diagnose, Treat, Monitor, and Eradicate Heart Attacks and Strokes While Growing Your Bottom Line

1st Edition. 2018

ASIN: B07DHZ3DWD (Amazon Kindle)

ISBN: 9781719976442 (Amazon Print)

ISBN: (Ingram Spark) PAPERBACK

ISBN: (Ingram Spark) HARDCOVER

ISBN: (Smashwords)

CONTACT THE AUTHOR:

Business Name: Todd C. Eldredge

Author Website: www.healthyheartco.com

LinkedIn:

Twitter:

Book Bonus:

Email:

Phone:

Cover design: Ry Stankeviciute

Library of Congress Cataloging-in-Publication Data

1. Medical books – Diseases - Cardiovascular.

2. Health, Fitness & Dieting – Diseases & Physical Ailments - Heart Disease

3. Medical Books – Administration & Policy - Health Risk Assessment

4. Medical Books - Internal Medicine - Cardiology

Printed in the United State of America

For Heidi – my soulmate and best friend.
You will always be my true north . . .

and for my Children, Grandchildren and my Parents . . .

you are ALL my happiest thoughts!

Testimonials

"I learned of CardioRisk and Todd Eldredge in 2009 at an advanced lipidology seminar at Saint Agnes Medical Center. I also obtained my first study at that time and became an immediate and avid supporter of CIMT and its implications in using an objective, highly reproducible study to assist in optimizing cardiovascular event reduction. It has been an invaluable component, and Todd has helped me to create a "cutting edge" preventative care practice.

I began my professional relationship and friendship with Todd shortly after that seminar. He is so incredibly knowledgeable and passionate about vascular disease and regularly, personally brings this to my office. Patients love his candor, knowledge and wonderful sense of humor. He is totally 'hands-on'!!

CIMT has helped me be a better preventative care physician and Todd Eldredge is the reason why!"

DR. TIMOTHY ROTH DO FAMILY MEDICINE

"Todd helped save my life with his knowledge, expertise, and experience. I was headed for a Cardiovascular Episode, but now I'm on the road to recovery & wellness."

TIM HARBOLT, DMD.

ABOUT THE AUTHOR

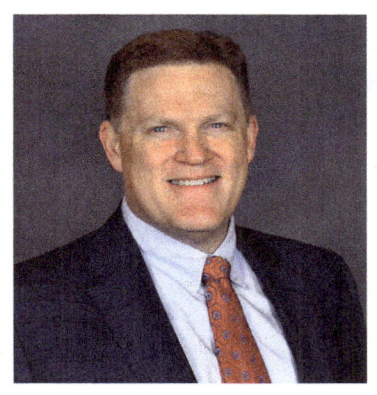

Todd Eldredge PhD, MPH, MBA Todd Eldredge is the Founder and Chief Executive Officer of CardioRisk Laboratories, an international heart attack, and stroke prevention company.

Eldredge co-founded the Wellness VIP (Vascular Improvement Program) (WellnessVIP, Inc.; www.wellnessvip.org) which integrates phenotypical, genotypical, and physical diagnostic testing to diagnose at-risk patients, optimize their care, and monitor the efficacy of treatment in patients with increased cardiovascular risk.

Prior to CardioRisk and WellnessVIP, Eldredge was a founder and/ or senior executive of several bio and technical companies with roots in quality, technology, and biologicals whose combined revenues exceeded $100MM in annual revenue. He helped to raise over $180MM in venture capital for these companies and he continues to consult for several technology based enterprises. Eldredge is a published best selling author and researcher and is involved in many CIMT-related research projects. Todd has spent many years developing performance-based testing protocols to demonstrate operator-dependent coefficients of variability and testing reproducibility. He spent 10 years at what is now Sanofi-Pasteur where he ran a Pediatric Vaccine Business Unit. Eldredge has a BSBA, MBA, and MPH degrees and a PhD in cardiovascular epidemiology.

PREFACE

Right now the medical world is broken! I can help!

The following story is about YOU! At least you should be able to see yourself or parts of yourself in this story . . . because this really is a story about YOU. It may not represent your life at this very minute . . . you may have moved on or made changes to fix the problem encapsulated in this very real story, but if you are or have ever been in the business of primary care medicine . . . then this story is about YOU. It is a story FOR you! I hope you can see yourself in the story.

Gerry is a good friend of mine. He is also a board-certified Internal Medicine physician. Over the years Gerry and I have had hundreds of conversations about life, about medicine, about what is happening to the practice of medicine, the effects of managed care and government sponsored health care, and what has happened to patient care.

Like many, Gerry went to medical school to make a difference. He romanticized the idea of being able to enhance and even preserve life. The idea of helping people to be well has been his most dominant thought. Making a lot of money never even entered his conscious mind.

This isn't to say he hadn't ever thought about money – he knew intuitively that physicians were well compensated and that the probability of starving or even having a lower middle-class income was remote – at least AFTER medical school. Money was just not something he needed to worry about.

Throughout medical school, rotations, residency, and now his own practice – the idea of helping people to be well was a primary concern. The secret thrill of listening to a patient's health concerns, having the ability to triage and categorize the range of possibilities and then knowing what to do about those concerns is unique to providers who have made the study of medicine their life's work.

Unfortunately, for many physicians, and more specifically, for Gerry, the practice of medicine has been relegated to the filling out of paperwork and forms, the entering of data into electronic medical health records systems (EHR), or chasing 3rd party payers to get paid . . . so much so that there is very little, if any, time for a personal life or time to pursue hobbies, other interests and/or talents.

The average Primary Care physician needs to see 30 – 50 patients every day just to pay their bills. When you see that many patients each day, the time to interact in a meaningful way just doesn't exist. The business of medicine has turned Primary Care providers into mini production factories and stripped many of them of the part of medicine they valued most . . . patient relationships. This trend has the effect of turning thousands away from the field of medicine. Thousands more are abandoning the traditional practice of medicine for concierge practices. This forces them to fire many of their patients to manage smaller groups of patients who pay for the 'privilege' of access to their provider.

Beyond that, medical malpractice has pushed providers like Gerry into the proverbial corner of standardized medicine which virtually every provider recognizes as the LOWEST standard of care, not something to be admired or desired by a patient. This 'no child left behind' of health care otherwise known as 'the standard of care', is getting people killed. Gerry once described the standard of care as the lowest standard of care allowed by law in order to avoid being sued for malpractice. The standard of care stands in direct contrast to what every provider WANTS to give their patients, and what most patients really desire . . . 'Optimal Care'. Optimal care, however, is rarely paid for by 3rd party payers. Optimal care requires out of pocket payment which offends our sense of fairness and even the belief of feasibility for many or most of our patients.

Is it any wonder why the United States' health care system has fallen to dead last out of 11 industrialized countries analyzed by the commonwealth fund (Mahon, 2017)? The Kaiser Family Foundation found that the disease burden in the US is significantly higher (23,104 per 100,000 of population) than any other industrialize or comparable country. The disease rate in the US is nearly 5,000 per 100,000 patients

HIGHER than the average of industrialized nations (Sawyer, 2017). According to the World Health Organization, which actively monitors 190 countries, the US ranks 37th and Canada 30th in terms of the quality of their health care systems (WHO, 2000). How does that happen? Well THAT will have to be the subject of a different book. The point here is that physicians like Gerry are feeling the pressure of a system that is failing them and it is failing their patients.

Just as important, however, is that this system is creating fatigue and dissatisfaction in the ranks of the nearly 200,000 Primary Care providers in the US. This has caused many of them to leave medicine altogether, to sell their practice to an HMO, hospital, or other corporate conglomerate, to leave practice and join the executive corporate management of a pharmaceutical., blood laboratory, or medical brain trust, or they just move into non-traditional pay-for-service models and give up a large number of their patients. The shortage of physicians anticipated in the next 10 years exceeds 100,000.

If you are one of these physicians, then this book was written for you and to you. I hope you will find hope and encouragement as you flip through its pages. This book won't attempt to solve all the problems presented to Primary Care providers – but it does solve a major one.

A full quarter of the deaths in the US are caused by a single disease – one which is nearly 100% preventable (Murphy, 2017). Were a similar number of deaths to be caused by car accidents, or gun violence, the world and the nation would be incensed. Somehow because it is a disease that most feel is just inevitable . . . it escapes our wrath. Think about it for just one second – nearly a full quarter of ALL deaths in the US are caused by one single, preventable disease.

This book will ask you to make just one, two, or three changes to your practice that will make an enormous impact on the health of your patient population. Yes – the evidence will show that making these changes will eradicate heart attacks and strokes, caused by atherosclerosis, from your practice. That may not save all your patients . . . after all, we know that death is unavoidable in the long-run. Imagine, however, the joy, happiness, and extra minutes of life and quality of life you can provide to your patients by making just a few simple and minor adjustments to the way you practice medicine.

The reward would be worth it even if there was no financial benefit to you or your practice. Having said that – these changes can also drive additional revenue and profit opportunities to your practice. I know, profit and revenue are nearly forbidden words in the language of medicine – but they do represent a fair exchange for the added playing time in the game of life you will provide to your patients.

When you finish reading these pages – I hope you will take action. After all – what good is the prescription you write for your patients if they don't ever fill it? No intervention will work unless and until it is implemented.

I wish you luck in your pursuit of excellence and your quest to find satisfaction and joy in one of the most important professions of our day. God bless you for your desire to help others.

With love, affection, and admiration.

-Todd-

HOW TO READ THIS BOOK:

Gestalt Theory learning suggests that learning happens best when the instruction is related to your own real-life experiences (David, 2015). Since this book is written for you – and I am writing directly to you, yes YOU . . . I am hopeful you will catch glimpses of yourself within its pages. When you do – then the solution prescribed between these pages can be absorbed and applied to your own situation via the Gestalt method.

For years I was a member of a group of business executives where as a small group of peers we attempted to make improvements to our own lives and businesses. The operational rules of engagement were based on the premise that if you told a peer what to do to solve their problems it was at once distasteful and threatening and would probably not be well received. Further – the other members of the group would call you out for doing so. It was one of the strictest rules of our Mastermind group. To violate this method of communication would suggest that one member or members of the forum thought they knew more than another member – which eviscerated the efficacy of the group.

Instead the forum utilized the Gestalt method which consisted of various members of the forum sharing their own experience of when they faced a similar situation, what they did about it, and how it turned out. The net effect of this methodology is that everyone in the forum could benefit, even though the response(s) were directed at a completely different and often unrelated situation.

Also, there is no reason to interpret each member's response as a threat to one's knowledge, masculinity/femininity, or business prowess since each member shares only the experience through their own eyes. It's almost impossible for you to effectively critique my experience as interpreted through my own eyes – or for me to critique yours. Each person shares their unique experience, and the uniqueness of their perspective allows each to share in a non-threatening way which enables all to enjoy and all to derive their own meaning. I can't tell you how useful that methodology was to me.

Over and over again I would hear stories shared by members of my own forum. These stories would often be completely unrelated to my business or circumstances. Nevertheless, these stories would consistently teach me some profound principle that did relate directly to my own situation. If you haven't participated in a MasterMind group, I highly recommend it.

It is my hope as you read through this book that you can apply the Gestaldt method of learning. Even though these stories might be about someone else – and may be only remotely related to your specific situation, see how these stories may relate to you, your practice, your patients, even if they don't completely match the details of your unique situation.

When I wrote this book, I had in mind a particular physician friend of mine. This helped me to direct my thoughts towards an individual rather than to a group. When you read this book, it would be good to think of me as your friend setting across your desk having a conversation with you about this horrific disease, rather than yourself as a student sitting in a classroom full of 300 other physicians listening to a professor. This will also serve to better explain the tone and voice of the text.

What you won't get in this book is the type of lecture you would find in a typical textbook. Yes, there will be the inevitable and expected levels of scientific research, but that research will be flavored by real-world experiences told by individuals affected by the disease. Medicine as a theoretical construct, is less valuable until it's practiced on 'the one'. Because of this perspective, I've included personal stories, which will help you understand better where I'm coming from and why this disease matters to me. I have always believed that when you understand someone's heart, you are better prepared to understand where they are coming from and any message they try to communicate.

TRAGEDY AND TRIUMPH – OR 'WHY I CARE'

While in my Freshman year of High School, my mind was occupied by many of the activities and curriculum that consume the thoughts of a typical 15-year-old young man. Sports; friends; scholarship . . . well, . . . not so much; girls . . . (definitely!); the movie coming out next month; music on the radio and more specifically, who would win Casey Kasem's top 40 this weekend; these were the types of ideas that occupied my mind as best as I can recall in the winter of 1977.

My mom and dad had six children. My younger brother Stephen died at birth leaving my parents with five otherwise healthy children. My older brother David and I had what I consider to be a typical sibling relationship. We quarreled, we fought, we even knocked each other out at one point, but within the confines of what I consider a typical sibling relationship was a deep and abiding love and friendship for each other that only two brothers separated by a few years of age can know or understand.

My parents owned a baby blue 1970 Chevy Kingswood Wagon – a station wagon with that famous Chevy 350 V-8 engine. It drank gas . . . at about 6MPG by the time I was driving it. This car has been relegated and assigned to the unfortunate position of being the primary family learning fleet vehicle, as it was the car designated for use by each of my siblings when we learned to drive. I say designated because it never really made it past my own experience . . . and I was #2 in the family birth order.

As the first sibling to reach the age of 16, David got to drive it first. He managed to put several dents in the car in the form of minor fender-benders, causing great consternation to those of us who had yet to matriculate through a proper driver's education course nor even reach a legal age in order to take it for a test drive.

One of the biggest arguments I had with my brother concerned his negligent driving habits and the affect those habits may have had on my future opportunity to drive, let alone my potential access to a functioning vehicle.

Having established that I was not yet old enough to drive legally, my primary mode of transportation was the city bus. My daily weekday routine consisted of arriving at the appropriate bus stop just in time, but not a minute too soon, to catch the scheduled route and arrive at my appointed destination in time to converse with friends who found themselves in a similar situation. Daily I dreamed and counted the days until I could at least share the family's vehicle with my brother, or, even better, until the day he left for college and I could inherit the asset entirely for my own enjoyment. Such was my station in life in February of 1977.

Upon arriving home on a Thursday afternoon of that year, I began my near religious weekday ritual of watching my favorite cartoons and sitcoms: Gilligan's Island, Batman, and the Flintstones were a few of my favorites. It's a bit sequacious to remind some that there was no Internet, iTunes, Netflix, and only a few channels of cable TV were available in 1977 – and we didn't have that luxury.

Somewhere during this standardized routine, a call came through the family phone (we also didn't have cell or wireless phones in those days – they were all corded phones). My mother answered and upon completion she casually explained that David had been in an accident and she had to go get him.

"Great", I remember thinking . . . "He's wrecked the car again". After all, we had been through this routine before . . . several times. I didn't give it too much more thought than that. However, as the sitcoms and cartoons continued long past my standard routine, and into the early evening, I became acutely aware of a nervous and foreboding feeling that had slowly crept into my conscience. By 6:00 PM it had fully taken center stage.

At length I realized that my parents had simply been gone for too long. As the minutes turned into hours, that sense of fear and foreboding increased, and genuine worry began to fill my mind as I openly acknowledged the concern I was trying desperately to ignore. What could possibly be taking my parents so long?

At length I heard the family car pulling up to the curb and the unmistakable sound of the car doors opening and closing. However, these somewhat routine sounds were accompanied by what, at first blush, sounded like a hideous laugh . . . I subsequently but quickly recognized it as the sound of my mother crying hysterically. "Trouble . . . big trouble" I thought.

I sprinted down the stairs of our home and out the front door, off the porch and down the cement stairs that led to porch where I was met by my parents. My Dad was practically carrying my Mother. I will never forget the painful expressions emoting from their long faces. As we met physically on the sidewalk my father was able to manage a broken whisper of despair and he said to me – "Son, . . . David is dead, . . . he was killed in a car accident."

Unless you have personally experienced something like this – there is no way to describe the weight or the impact of those words. A kick in the gut doesn't begin to properly describe the sensation – though they would be in the correct quadrant of pain. The words alone literally knocked me off my feet and I fell to my knees in shock and despair as my mind grasped for meaning and I tried in vain to wrap my young mind around what it meant. Truthfully, it would take years to process.

There simply are no words to describe the sudden and tragic loss of life of a family member. Though millions have gone through similar events, and many millions more will undoubtedly experience similar emotions . . . my experience was unique to me . . . as I'm sure their experiences are completely, and unequivocally unique to them.

There was nothing I nor anyone else could have done to prevent this tragedy. My brother was a passenger in a car driven by someone else, along with 5 of his friends. The truck that ran into them, full of salty sand to spread on the slippery streets of our snow-covered city, was also driven by a well-intentioned driver.

I suppose it is a natural element of any disaster to attempt to assign blame . . . I mean, how could this possibly happen? What could have been done differently? At the end of the day, there are no real answers to those questions . . . and even if there were, I'm not sure it would bring any comfort to those who mourn the loss of a loved one.

For me – this experience is one of several which shape and inform many of the thoughts, feelings, and motivations I have relating to the sanctity and value of life, the importance of telling people we love them, and of sharing what they mean to us, and how paramount it is to treasure time with loved ones . . . because we simply never know when the fragility of life will tip the scales and those we care deeply about will disappear from this realm we can see and touch.

Now please don't think after reading this that I am a mere sentimentalist. I am also a realist who embraces science and scientific method. I've read the book of life, and I understand it is a tragic love story. I mean . . . we all know how it ends. Spoiler alert: None of us are getting out of this alive.

Having said that, I also believe that it is noble and meritorious to engage in those activities that extend the quality and quantity of life. Even though the ending is inevitable . . . the importance of being able to write a better . . . more prolonged . . . happier ending cannot be understated. As my physician friend Gerry put it: "We are engaged in the art of adding play time minutes to the game of life". I love that!

In the case of my older brother, there was literally nothing that I could have done that would have altered his ending. This is tragic – but I can accept it as a metaphysical certainty.

By now I can imagine you must be thinking, "yes, but what does this have to do with the price of beans in China" . . . or more specifically, "what does it have to do with Heart attack and Stroke prevention?"

Let's fast forward a few decades to bring this discussion full circle. Contextual meaning is relevant to understanding where people are coming from . . . this backdrop should shed additional light on why all this matters, or at least why it matters to me.

As a function of my education and professional associations I became acquainted with technology that showed promise in its ability to identify those at increased risk for Heart Attacks and Strokes in time to treat their disease medically, instead of waiting until it had to be treated surgically. I was aware that many people never make it or get the opportunity to qualify for a surgical intervention because the first sign or symptom they had was a massive heart attack or stroke. Over half of those, whose first symptom was the heart attack or stroke, die from that event. Waiting for signs, symptoms, or enough arterial obstruction to provide ethical justification for the Cardiologist or Vascular Surgeon to intervene surgically is just not a rational option. For most of the population, prevention is the only viable and reliable option. If we want to put a dent in the current morbidity and mortality statistics owing to cardiovascular disease, then we must do a much better job of identifying this expanding universe of people at risk for disease and events, and we then need to take aggressive prescriptive action to intervene and stop the progression of this disease and its sequelae. The earlier we can take action, the more likely it is we can preserve and enhance human life.

I was enthralled with this technology from the very first minute I was exposed to it. I was surprised at the vast amount of research that had already been published by the time I was introduced. I couldn't contain my enthusiasm or curiosity to better understand this technology.

At length I was able to receive one-on-one training from one of the men who pioneered the method, Dr. Gene Bond. Dr. Bond is one of the most knowledgeable people I ever met on any subject. He is especially gifted with regards to his knowledge about atherosclerosis and other arterial diseases, the tools used to image and assess the disease, its etiology and pathophysiological pathways. Dr. Bond's curriculum vitae is a book in and of itself. It took me nearly 5 years of concerted effort just to read through and absorb the volumes of his published research. Dr. Bond was a co-author of the Atherosclerosis Risk In Community (ARIC) and many other landmark epidemiologic studies. He had been a professor of medicine at Wake Forest school of medicine for nearly 30 years. He was a gifted pathologist with a masters in anatomy. It was a highlight of my life to have been mentored by him and to have spent nearly 10 years learning from his experience. To be truthful, it is unlikely I will ever know everything Dr. Bond knew about this disease – but one hopes that one has at least understood the most crucial and important details uncovered during the time I was fortunate enough to have spent by his side. Beyond that, and somewhat parenthetically, Dr. Bond is a compassionate, kind, and caring human being who was a gentleman in every human interaction I ever witnessed.

Sometime during my training, and after having demonstrated proficiency of the method via a double-blind, performance-based certification, I took an ultrasound machine with me to my parent's home for a Thanksgiving holiday. I was anxious to share some of my knowledge about this technology, and I was anxious to demonstrate for my siblings that they were all healthy. I expected nothing less. My family were supportive of my enthusiasm and each agreed to let me examine their carotids.

My next younger brother is 7 years younger. He is a commercial airline pilot. In my mind, he was the picture of health. At the time of my first scan of his arteries, he was running around 5 miles each day, usually at least 5 days each week. He didn't have a stitch of fat on his body. He was tall and slender and seemed to have a relatively stress-free life (easy for me to say.) Upon beginning the ultrasonic mapping process of his arteries my eyes caught a glimpse of something that had my full attention. Closer examination confirmed what my mind could not conceive. I simply could not wrap my head around this . . . but there it was . . . a large, eccentric, echoluscent or soft atherosclerotic plaque in his right carotid artery. A widow-maker. I instantly understood the ramifications of this lesion. Research told me that approximately 82% of the lesions this size were likely to rupture in a 10-year window if left untreated. Additional research told me that this lipid-rich plaque was 11 times more likely to rupture than a similarly sized echogenic plaque and I remember feeling that same sense of foreboding and dread I had experienced while waiting to hear about my older brother's condition.

I simply couldn't bear the thought of prematurely losing another sibling – especially via a disease that was nearly 100% preventable. Not on MY WATCH!

To make a long story short – I was able to get my brother connected with an expert in treating this disease and preventing potential events. I made arrangements with Dr's Amy Doneen and Bradley Bale (of the Bale/Doneen Method, and the Heart Attack and Stroke Prevention Center in Spokane, WA.) and Amy was kind enough to see my brother and begin treating him almost immediately.

At the time of this book's publication, it's been well over a decade since I first found this lesion in my brother's artery. He still flies commercially. He has raised his two children to adulthood. He has weathered the stressful storms I've subsequently learned are inherent in commercial aviation (buyouts, furloughs, working abroad) and has managed to stay healthy and free from even the slightest sign or symptom of cardiovascular disease. As a caveat of his treatment, he is no longer pre-diabetic, and it is highly likely he will live a long and prosperous life. There is no question that Dr. Doneen added playing time to his game of life. Although his end is imminent (as it is for us all) – it is unlikely that his final demise will be related to cardiovascular disease.

To me this last story underscores the reality of the disease – it is not just a case study for those who are touched by its reach. To those affected by its insidious tentacles, the disease is real. This disease impacts real people, real jobs, real families, and it affects real incomes. It is not merely a case study that we listen to in an auditorium full of medical or graduate students. I cannot detach myself from the familial aspects and its heightened potential for emotional impact.

Although I was unable to do anything about my older brother's death. I was, and I am able to do something about the lives of friends, families, and acquaintances of contact to help extend the quality and quantity of their lives. These two events (two brother's lives) motivate me every single day. These stories keep the disease at the forefront of my thoughts and they are consummate reminders that 'this' (disease prevention) matters. This disease has affected my parents, my siblings, aunts, uncles, cousins, and many other friends and family. It has also touched me in a very personal way, as my own arteries needed aggressive therapy.

I think without looking too far, you will find this disease is rampant. You will not have to pay too close attention or look very far into your own sphere of influence to find it is affecting your own friends and family, not to mention the patients who count on your vigilance on their behalf. Just about everyone with whom I come in contact personally knows of someone in their forties, or fifties and even younger who keeled over unexpectedly from a massive heart attack or stroke.

For the most part, these events are nearly 100% preventable. When I first began studying this disease it was responsible for over half the deaths. Think about that for a minute - nearly one half of all deaths were related to a single, largely preventable, disease. Statins and stents have had a significant impact on the morbidity and mortality of the disease. Further progress may be hindered, however, unless and until the medical community gets more effective at identifying those at risk earlier and subsequently providing them with appropriate treatment before patients need surgical interventions. Absent those interventions, this disease will continue to take life unnecessarily, and unexpectedly. Today this disease is responsible for closer to 1 in every 4 deaths (CDC, 2018). When one stops to consider that most of these deaths are preventable . . . we simply cannot afford to become complacent.

In the chapters that follow, this book addresses simple strategies which will help physician' to better identify those at increased risk, prescribe appropriate interventions, and monitor the efficacy of that prescribed treatment. Only then can we be certain we have, in fact, derailed the disease and removed it from the leading causes of death in North and South America.

THE DISEASE – AND . . . SOME SCIENCE

According to the World Health Organization (WHO), Heart Attacks and Strokes are the number one leading cause of death worldwide. Coronary Artery Disease and Stroke collectively account for more than the next three leading causes of death combined, and they are responsible for over 15 Million deaths each year. Sadly, most of these events are nearly completely preventable.

The US healthcare system encourages and rewards treatments and procedures over prevention and outcomes. Experts agree that this is at least partially responsible for the country's slip to 37th place among 190 industrialized nations in terms of key health outcomes. The standard of care in the US compels physicians to identify and treat risk factors rather than disease. This approach results in Heart Attacks and Strokes accounting for nearly one third of all deaths in the US, and more in the rest of the world (Murphy, 2017).

In the United States, someone has a heart attack approximately every 34 seconds. Someone dies from one every minute (Go, 2014).

Stroke is still the number one cause of disability. Someone has a stroke every 40 seconds in the United States. Someone dies from a stroke every four minutes (Falk, 1995)[i]. In 2007 alone, over 150,000 of those deaths were from patients who were younger than 65.

Over 70 percent of those clinical events (heart attacks and strokes) have a single disease at the root of their collective tree. That root (atherosclerosis) is nearly 100% preventable.

Oh – and as we discussed earlier, but on the outside chance your eyes glazed over that part . . . nearly one out of three deaths are caused by this insidious disease (Murphy, 2017). I can't help but hammer that one home.

The audacity and complacency necessary to allow any single and largely preventable phenomenon to continue to take that many people off our fair planet is beyond me. I mean, we've sent men to the moon for God's sake! How in the world can we allow this Machiavellian infirmity to continue to wreak havoc on the populations of the world? Susan Powter said it best . . . (even if she wasn't referring to heart disease) "Stop the insanity"

Death's not so bad you say? I mean, after all, we all have to go sometime . . . right? Yes – that's true, and without waxing eloquent in philosophical or metaphysical discussions about whether it is meritorious or not to preserve life, let's just table the death sentence this disease imposes on a full third of our population and focus instead on its sequelae.

Four million people each year report disability from heart attack and stroke. That's right, many people say 'if I gotta go, I'd rather go from a heart attack', the problem with that philosophy is two fold: 1) You don't HAVE to go that early. 2) You can't be certain you will die from the event . . . you may just wake up and find that you need your children to change your diapers. Dying from the disease is one thing . . . but living in a miserable condition where you have no quality of life is quite another.

Then there is the element of cost. Kaiser Permanente performed a study in their closed system several years ago and determined that the average cost for a single day's stay for patients who had experienced a heart attack was approaching $55,000. The average length of stay for these patients was 5 days. The total **annual** estimated impact to the US healthcare system in terms of both direct and indirect costs exceeds $315 Billion, and it is expected to top $1.2 Trillion by the year 2030.

There is simply no acceptable answer for continuing to allow this disease to have the effect on the quality and quantity of life that it has. Frankly, there is really no excuse for its continued existence as a top 10 leading cause of death and disability.

Atherosclerosis – the Disease

Atherosclerosis, (from the Greek roots Athēra meaning 'Artery' and *sklēros*, meaning 'hardening' or 'scarring'), is responsible for the vast majority of clinical cardio and cerebrovascular events. Did I mention it is nearly 100% preventable?

At its most basic level, Atherosclerosis is a disease which is not at all unlike acne. Contrary to a very popular belief, it is not like a plumbing pipe that gets lined with residue over time.

The reason that most heart attacks and strokes are sudden and spontaneous is nefarious. How many times have you heard of someone calling in sick for work because they were 'coming down with a stroke'? How about 'never'?! Heart attack and strokes don't work like that.

The reason these events are sudden and spontaneous (in most cases) is that these lesions (called plaques and which are analogous to acne pimples) rupture. When they rupture one of two things happen: 1) the necrotic puss-like material in the plaque is pushed to the smaller vessels of the brain until they can move no further. Or 2) Upon rupture, enzymes are released into the blood stream which activate platelets in the blood signaling to them to begin healing the ruptured lesion via a scab. This creates a blood clot or thrombus which very often leads to the complete or partial blockage of blood flow.

At the end of the day, it doesn't matter whether the material in the necrotic core of the plaque causes the blockage, or the subsequent thrombus – either condition leads to potentially deadly series of events which result in either the brain or the heart starving for blood and/or oxygen.

A deeper dive into the disease reveals it is a chronic inflammatory disease which begins in the blood from pathogens that are carried throughout the vasculature and which eventually penetrate the thin one-cell thick layer which protects the rest of the arterial wall, the endothelium. Upon penetration into the inner layers of the arterial wall, the pathogens attract monocytes, which of course are floating around in the white blood cells. These monocytes then also penetrate the endothelium and into the inner layers of the arterial wall. At this point, the monocytes are activated and become macrophages. To keep this simple right now, we won't address the proliferation of adhesion molecules, cytokines, and the increased production of white blood cells – but the activated macrophages begin the disease elimination process called phagocytosis.

Phagocytosis is when the macrophages essentially consume these invading pathogens. Since they don't have a mechanism to make them stop eating, they eat until they literally explode. The byproducts of this consumption process are fatty steaks and foam cells, oxidized LDL which lead to inflammation and eventual eruption of a plaque lesion into the lumen of the vessel. This process is not at all unlike the formation of an acne lesion on the epidermis.

The wall of the artery heats up in response to the inflammatory response taking place inside the wall of the artery. Left untreated, this inflammation will eventually boil to the surface in the form of a plaque lesion which again, is not at all dissimilar to an acne pimple.

Athersclerosis – A Deeper Dive

Endothelial dysfunction in atherosclerosis involves a series of early changes that precede lesion formation. These changes include increased permeability of the lipoproteins and the upregulation of leukocyte (monocyte cells) and endothelial adhesion molecules. Subsequent to this upregulation, we see migration of the leukocytes into the arterial wall. During this initial phase of disease development, LDL-C accumulates in the subendothelial extracellular space within the wall of the artery (Solutions, 2005). (Figure 1)

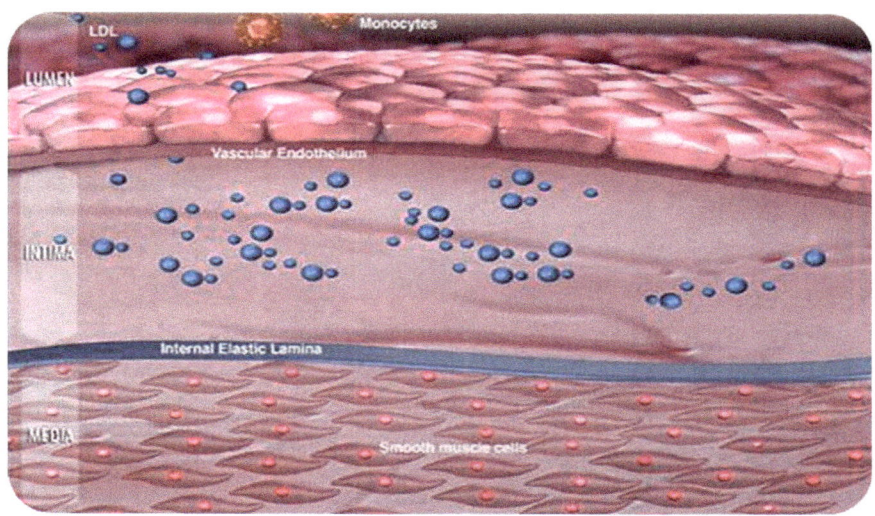

Figure 1

The local vascular cells of the endothelium mildly oxidize the LDL accumulated or trapped in the subendothelial extracellular space to form a minimally modified LDL which is then able to engage the recruitment of more monocytes and the eventual transition and deposition of macrophages. The macrophages continue to oxidize the LDL which has accumulated beneath the endothelium into the subendothelial extracellular space of the intima, to a form which can be eaten, scavenged, and internalized, resulting in the formation of foam cells. Foam cells represent the earliest lesion of atherosclerosis and can easily be detected by the thickening of the intima-media layers of the artery wall via B-mode ultrasound (Solutions, 2005). (Figure 2).

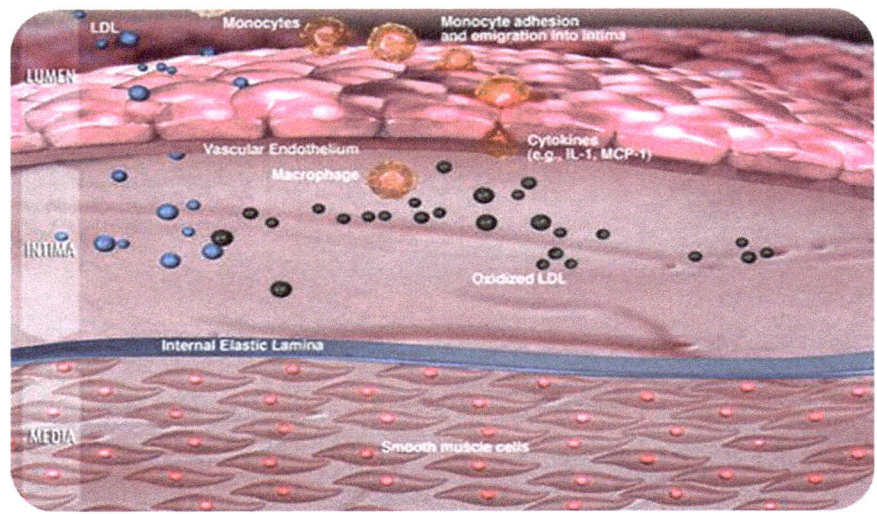

Figure 2

Fatty streak formation in atherosclerosis occurs when lipid-laden monocytes and macrophages along with T lymphocytes fail to filtrate and get trapped inside the wall of the artery. Later lesions include the invasion of smooth muscle tissue or the media layer of the artery. A complicated cascade of events follows which include migration into the smooth muscle tissue, T-cell activation, foam cell formation, and the adherence of platelets and their subsequent aggregation (Solutions, 2005). (Figure 3)

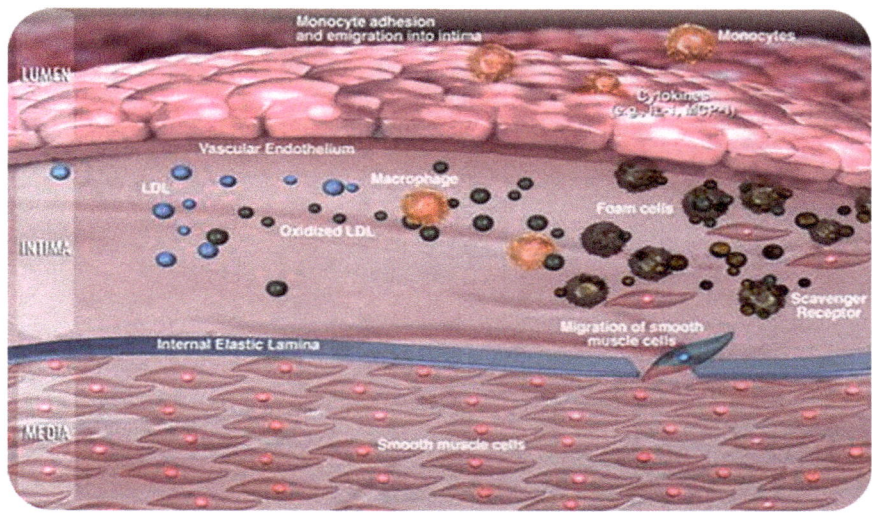

Figure 3

Formation of advanced atherosclerotic lesions begins initially with the development of a thin fibrous cap which creates a barrier between the lesion and the lumen of the artery. Leukocytes, lipids, and debris localize beneath this fibrous cap forming a necrotic core or soft plaque. The soft plaques are extremely vulnerable to rupture either through erosion, or via the increased pressure of blood flow through an increasingly narrowed vessel. Arterial plaques develop slowly, leading to the formation of lesions with a centralized lipid-rich core. This core contains many lipid-rich macrophage foam cells which are byproducts of the circulating monocyte activation and subsequent phagocytic process. As more monocytes pass through the arterial wall and become lipid-rich macrophages, they produce tissue factor, which is a potent coagulant. This glycoprotein activates an enzyme (Factor X) which is a protein family known as the cytokine receptor class II family. These enzymes promote or contribute to thrombogenicity of plaques adding to their vulnerability and potential for harm (Solutions, 2005). (Figure 4).

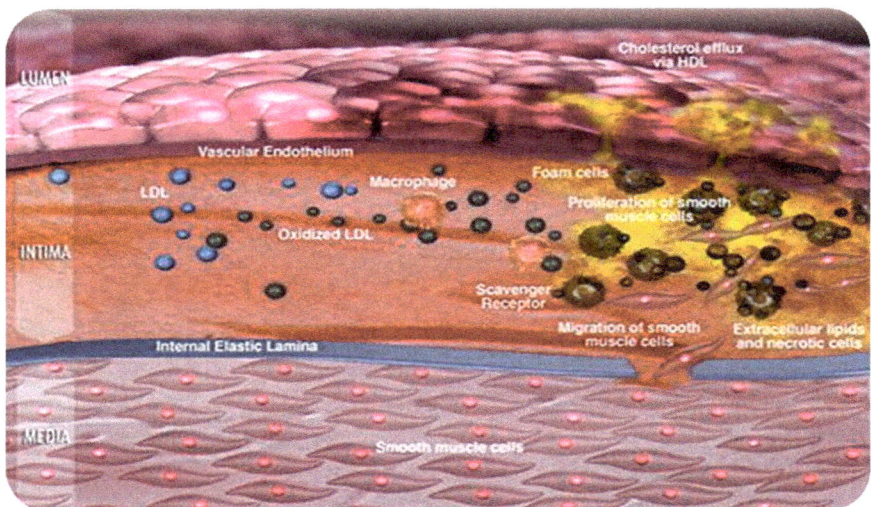

Figure 4

The development of a strong fibrous cap is the final phase of the disease and protects tissue factor and other cell matrix elements from escaping into the lumen and promoting thrombus formation. Minerals such as calcium form on the outer wall of the lesion providing additional stability and protection from rupture.

The reason that most heart attacks and strokes are sudden and spontaneous is because these lesions rupture. When they rupture, they do so suddenly and spontaneously.

As already discussed, rupture of plaque leads to a cascade of events including the release of enzymes into the blood stream which activate the platelets in the blood. These enzymes tell the platelets they need to begin the healing process and so the blood begins to form a scab proximate to the site of the rupture. A scab on the inside of an artery is, of course, deadly. A full 75% of the sudden deaths from Heart Attack are the direct result of a ruptured plaque (Kramer, 2010). So, we know that the white necrotic material of the plaque itself can cause a blockage, but often times it is the subsequent thrombus which causes the most damage.

Once again, at the end of the day, it doesn't really matter which of the two conditions causes the blockage – they are both deadly and can cause symptoms which lead to disability and or death. A significant point that should not be lost on this process.

For nearly 68% of those who experience a clinical event, their first sign or symptom was the heart attack or stroke itself (Falk, 1995). This means they didn't get the luxury of having signs and symptoms (chest pain, numbing of the arm, angina, etc). Half of those whose first sign or symptom was the event itself, die from this event. Think about that – for the majority of those who have a heart attack or stroke, they have very little if any blockage minutes or hours before their event. Their heart attack or stroke came on suddenly and spontaneously with virtually no warning in the form of signs and/or symptoms.

Given this pathophysiology, and the sudden and spontaneous presentation of clinical events, how can one more effectively go about the business of prevention?

The standard of care suggests the use of traditional risk factors. We won't rehash these well thought out strategies . . .except to say that they clearly are not enough. The title of this book suggests a 3-step plan which can significantly improve the event rate in your own practice. Let us now explore those modalities.

THE THREE STEP PROCESS:

Structure

Function

Blood

BLOOD –

Tim is a board-certified family physician friend of mine. We talk often as our children are of similar ages and stages of life. One of the reasons Tim went into medicine was not just to be able to diagnose disease and treat the risk factors, but he wanted to be able to treat the disease and improve health outcomes. One of the things that always amazes him is the fact that more physicians don't actively monitor and treat the actual disease. He feels they just monitor and treat the risk factors FOR disease. This drives him nuts!

In my mind there is relatively little or no value in having another book on the shelf that reviews once again (ad nauseum) the traditional blood bio monitors that together constitute the standard of care. I will, however, throw some data out there you may not be familiar with – not with any intention of discouraging you from continuing to utilize these tests and procedures, but to emphasize the need for caution. My intent is merely to make it clear that if you want to make a real difference . . . if you are tired of your patients reporting back to you they suffered a heart attack or stroke, then you have to consider changing a few things.

Many or even most primary care physicians make it their practice to screen their patients for abnormal blood values (e.g. risk factors for disease). As it relates to cardiovascular disease, and cardiovascular disease risk, physicians use some combination of Framingham Risk Score, or other metrics which provide loose guidance on their patient's future risk based on population health monitoring.

Total cholesterol, HDL cholesterol, and LDL cholesterol levels have been flagged as important prognostic data points in virtually all cardiovascular risk assessments. Indeed, the ATP III guidelines suggest that LDL cholesterol is or should be the primary target of therapy (Grundy, 2001). In a 2016 update – they suggest a "treat-to-target" guideline which varies depending on the patient's individual Framingham 10-year risk score.

To be fair, I have no intention on picking a fight with cholesterol (Total, LDL, HDL, or any sub fractionation of lipids). I do want to illustrate this point: If cholesterol screening and Framingham Risk Calculation represents the total extent of your risk stratification for your patients . . . your patients will continue to experience heart attacks and strokes.

Let's just review a couple of studies that underscore this point. Perhaps most damning was a study of 222 patients with no prior history of MI or CAD, lying in their bed subsequent to having experienced a recent acute myocardial infarction (Akosah, 2003). So – it's important to note that there was no question about whether or not the cohort in this study had active cardiovascular disease.

The authors then tested each of the patients' cholesterol levels and found the following: Only 18% of the women in the study, and 25% of the men qualified for a pharmacological intervention based on the current ATP III guidelines.

Think about that for a second – when looking at patients through the lens of the Framingham 10-year risk score, over ¾ of the patients who had been hospitalized for a heart attack, did not even qualify for pharmacological intervention. YIKES! If that number doesn't horrify you . . . I'm not sure what will.

Let's continue: Dr. Paul Ridker, a well-known professor of medicine at Harvard Medical School, and the Director of the Center for Cardiovascular Disease Prevention at Brigham and Women's Hospital, conducted a large study which involved Cholesterol as a screening tool (Ridker, 2002).

They looked at 27,939 apparently healthy American women and followed these women for a mean of eight years for cardio and cerebrovascular events. Now for the shocker: 77% of all events occurred among women whose LDL levels where below those recommended for treatment using the ATP III guidelines. 46% of the events occurred among patients whose LDL cholesterol levels were below 130 mg per deciliter. In other words – events are taking place every day in patients whose cholesterol levels are NORMAL! Not just SOME patients . . . but the MAJORITY of patients!

One more study, and then I'll let this go. This study of 136,905 patients hospitalized with CAD revealed that 77% of those patients had LDL levels below 130 mg/dl (Sachdeva A. C., 2009). They had NORMAL LDL cholesterol levels. In this large cohort of patients hospitalized with CAD, almost half had admission LDL levels below 100 mg/dL. 45.4% of these hospitalized patients had normal HDL levels above 40 mg/dL and 61.8% had normal triglyceride levels below 150 mg/dL.

All this spells trouble for any provider who look at lipids as their primary screening tool. These three data points underscore the issue that cholesterol testing alone is grossly inadequate at predicting who will and who will not go on to experience a cardiovascular event.

The reasons should be obvious. At the time that the phlebotomist sticks their needle into your patient's vein to extract a sample, not one drop of that blood has hurt your patient. At the very best the sample will tell us the quantity of a pathogen per deciliter of blood which will suggest a propensity or probability of causing problems in the future. Let us be clear though . . . at the time that the blood level is drawn, not one DROP of that drawn blood has hurt the patient. By definition, that blood was floating around in the circulatory of your patient seconds before it was drawn into a vial.

In order for those pathogens to cause damage to your patient . . . they must penetrate the wall of an organ, or a vessel. They simply cannot hurt you whilst floating around your circulatory.

This isn't to suggest that blood tests are not useful. You know that's not true. Of course, they are useful! Cholesterol explains nearly 50% of the disease. Cholesterol and lipid testing may be far more utile in defining treatment therapies, than in stratifying who is and who is not likely to experience a future event.

What we are suggesting is that if this (cholesterol testing) is the extent of your risk assessment . . . and especially if that assessment is only done at an annual visit, you will continue to lose patients prematurely.

The evidence can be found in the most recent epidemiologic statistics on cardio and cerebrovascular disease (Murphy, 2017).

At the end of the day, these diseases still cause as many deaths as the next three leading causes of death combined, and they account for nearly one third of the deaths in the US. That is simply unacceptable.

Still we cannot take our eyes off the patient's blood work. It is in the blood that we find clues as to what may be causing inflammation, and whether or not treatment has been effective.

It was never this book's intent to provide a comprehensive look at all biomarker testing you could be using to more effectively stratify risk in your patients. Having said that, there are a few blood/bio tests you may not have considered, which could enhance your cardiovascular risk assessment prowess.

For a more comprehensive list of *Red Flags* or cardiovascular risk assessments, AND THEIR TREATMENTS, may I strongly recommend to you a book and preceptorship by two friends who have made heart attack and stroke prevention their life's work. One of the things that separates them from any other provider I know is that they provide a written guarantee. That's right – a guarantee! If one of their patients has a heart attack and/or stroke. . . they give back 100% of the medical fees that patient paid during the year. That is something you don't see very much of in this litigious world of healthcare we find ourselves in. So write this down, the book is *"Beat the Heart Attack Gene"* by Dr's Bradley Bale, MD, and Amy Doneen, DNP. If you don't have this on your current bookshelf, stop now and order it! **https:www.baledoneen.com**

In the meantime, here are a few bio monitors that if you are not already using, you may want to consider:

Fibrinogen – this analyte measures the amount of a glycoprotein in your blood. It is a soluble, sticky, fibrous protein produced in the liver which helps to stop excessive bleeding via blood clots. When certain enzymes are released into the blood stream following a vascular injury such as a plaque rupture, thrombin is enzymatically converted to fibrin, to form a fibrin-based blood clot. When a patient has too much Fibrinogen, it can point to a potential risk of blood clots and a cascade of other events which lead to cardio and cerebrovascular events.

Microalbumin/Creatinine – Microalbumin is a blood protein found in the urine. Virtually no albumin is present in the urine when kidneys are functioning properly. Protein in the urine is abnormal and albumin is a large protein molecule that circulates in the blood. If it leaks from the capillaries in the kidneys into the urine, we know that endothelial dysfunction is highly likely. We'll discuss endothelial function and dysfunction more thoroughly in another chapter. The short version is that whenever there is endothelial dysfunction, the risk for coronary and cerebrovascular events is significantly increased.

The ratio comes from measuring the amounts of microalbumin with those of creatinine. Creatinine is a chemical waste molecule generated from muscle metabolism. Very few providers (in my experience) use it regularly because it is most commonly used to screen people with diabetes, high blood pressure, or kidney disorders. It is, however, an independent biomarker that predicts risk for cardiovascular events. People with elevated MACR had a 20 percent higher rate of CV events, even when other risk factors were considered. It is an inexpensive test and is generally covered by 3rd party payers.

Lp-PLA2 – Lipoprotein-Associated Phospholipase A-2. - This test is also known as a platelet-activating factor acetyl hydrolase (PAF-AH). This test measures an enzyme that appears to play a role in the inflammation of blood vessels and is thought to promote atherosclerosis. The enzyme is associated with disease activity within the wall of the artery and, most importantly, the activity below the collagen or calcified cap caused by active phagocytic activity of active macrophages. Lp-PLA2 interacts with oxidized LDL to increase inflammation and increase the atherogenic state. This, in turn, leads to increased risk of plaque vulnerability. This test is especially useful in conjunction with a CIMT test. If plaque is found in the arterial wall, Lp-PLA2 could imply higher and more immediate risk (Goncalves, 2012) of future plaque rupture.

Myeloperoxidase (MPO) - A peroxidase enzyme that is most abundantly expressed in white blood cells, and which produces hypothallus and hypochlorous acids to carry out antimicrobial activity. In other words, the human immune system uses MPO to fight infection. It has been implicated in various types of vasculitis, and other disorders that destroy blood vessels via inflammation in the arteries. One study reported that elevated MPO levels more than doubled the risk for cardiovascular mortality over a 13-year period (Heslop, 2010).

MPO reduces the production of nitric oxide (NO), a key signaling molecule, leading to vasodilation and many physiological and pathological processes. NO is a key component in vascular function – so decreased production of NO is a risk factor by itself. When MPO is elevated or too high, it makes ALL cholesterol compounds more inflammatory (even HDL). This enzyme can produce hypochlorous acid (by interacting with hydrogen peroxide) in the blood stream which eats a hole in the thin layer protecting the inner wall of the artery (the endothelium) allowing easier access for even small amounts of cholesterol. MPO is dangerous in that it produces numerous oxidants – all of them bad for the arteries.

ApoB - The primary apolipoprotein of the chylomicrons responsible for carrying fat molecules or lipids (including cholesterol) around the body to all cells within all tissues. ApoB is the primary protein which organizes the particles and is essential to the formation of these fat particles. The ApoB serves as a ligand or binding molecule for LDL receptors. This means that it signals that the particles containing fat are ready to enter those cells with ApoB receptors and thus deliver the fats into the other cells of the body.

High levels of ApoB are the primary driver of plaque in the arterial wall, which are the primary cause of vascular disease or atherosclerosis. In an 8-year prospective study of 9231 asymptomatic women and men from the Danish general population, patients with elevated ApoB (top tertile vs. bottom tertile) had an 80% - 140% higher hazard ratio for any ischemic cardiovascular event. ApoB had a higher predictive ability than did LDL cholesterol in the prediction of ischemic heart disease, myocardial infarction, and any ischemic cardiovascular event in both genders (Benn, 2006).

LP(a) – A genetic, sticky, fatty, lipoprotein particle found in the blood. The apolipoprotein(a) is covalently bound to the ApoB particle. Elevated LP(a) concentrations are highly heritable. Although the association is stronger between Lp(a) and cardiovascular disease than it is to stroke, it is predictive of both. Niacin (Vitamin B3) has been proven effective at reducing levels of LP(a).

LP(a) accumulates in the vessel wall and inhibits the binding of PLG, suggesting that it generates blood clots and atherosclerosis. In meta-analysis of the cohort studies looking at the relationship between LP(a) and stroke, the risk ratio was 22% higher for stroke in patients with elevated LP(a) (Smolders, 2007). A separate meta-analysis of 18 major prospective studies showed a 70% increase in the combined risk ratio of patients in the top tertile vs. bottom tertile of LP(a) blood concentrations (Danesh, 2018).

F2 Isoprostanes – This urine test is a direct measure and the gold standard to quantify lipid peroxidation/oxidative stress in vivo. These prostaglandin-like compounds are key factors in the creation of oxidative stress. Oxidative stress results from the generation and an overaccumulation of reactive oxygen and nitrogen. It represents an imbalance between the formation of antioxidant defenses (a good thing) and the formation of free radicals (a bad thing).

Increased oxidative stress leads to premature aging, the development of cancer, and of course, cardiovascular disease. This accumulation of F2 Isoprostanes has been shown to damage lipoproteins, lipids, DNA, and other proteins. The modification of these lipoproteins and DNA can lead to the alteration of endothelial function and inflammatory processes which result in the progression of atherosclerosis and cardiovascular disease. F2-Isoprostanes may increase aspirin resistance to platelet aggregation within platelets and whole blood. In short – elevated F2-Isoprostane reflects widespread oxidative stress and systemic burden of lipid peroxidation end products. This biomarker is a direct reflection of a patient's lifestyle and, in fact, is best treated by positive changes in lifestyle management. Since there is not a pill made that is more effective that positive lifestyle management . . . it is an important bio monitor and the 'truth serum' of effective lifestyle management.

Genetic Tests – There are a few genetic tests you may want to consider as well. Genetic tests are economical, because they never change. You only do genetic tests once in a lifetime. Also, they provide unique insight into certain genetic predispositions. Here are a few you may want to consider:

9P21 Genotype – About 25% of Caucasians and Asians are homozygous for 9P21. This means they have inherited the gene from their mother and father. If you are positive for this gene (e.g. you are a carrier)– you have 102% rise in risk for heart attack and/or stroke at an early age compared to non-carriers of the gene. Your lifetime risk increases by 56%. Your risk would be much higher for severe coronary artery disease affecting multiple arteries – and you have about a 74% increased risk for aortic abdominal aneurysm. About 50% of the Caucasian and Asian population are heterozygous – meaning they inherited only one copy of the gene inherited from EITHER their father or mother. This group have ½ the risks found in the homozygous carriers – but still elevated significantly. These risks were independent of other risk factors such as family history, diabetes, high blood pressure, and elevated inflammatory markers, and even obesity – so it's an important test.

ApoE – This is a gene type which influences lifetime risk of coronary heart disease and Alzheimer's – it also provides unique insight as to how your body metabolizes nutrients in your diet (including both fats and carbs). Just as an example, it your patient had a 2-4, a 3-4, or a 4-4 profile, their lifetime risk for CVD is significantly increased. This group could trim the threat of risk by following a low-fat diet (no more than 20%) and by limiting or completely avoiding alcohol as they don't metabolize it very effectively. Metabolic advice is available for every ApoE genotype and this direction is useful for both ideal weight management as well as cardiovascular risk reduction.

Interleukins – Interleukins are genetic variants linked to heightened response to inflammation. Since these genes are among the first to be activated during the body's inflammatory response (a disease prevention mechanism) they ignite a chain reaction leading to the release of other chemicals in the body. When these chemicals are released at a higher-than-normal level to escalate and sustain the body' response to disease – additional problems are imminent. This makes patients more prone to chronic inflammation and a more intense acute response than we like. So – these interleukins lay dormant until challenged – but when the body is challenged with a pathogen, they respond more severely than is needed . . . causing damage to important structures like the arterial wall. Elevated levels of Interleukins indicate potential trouble in the walls of the arteries.

Oral Hygiene – All humans harbor literally millions of bacteria in their mouths. Some of them are crucial to digestion and good health. Two of them are not beneficial at all and, in fact, are causative of cardiovascular disease. A fairly recent study published in conjunction with Johns Hopkins university found that two specific bacteria found in the mouth were causative of cardiovascular disease (Bale, 2016). If your patients never have bleeding gums and have had no prior evidence of periodontal disease, they probably do not need an oral DNA test – however, if either of those conditions exist . . . including if they have ever had periodontal disease, they will have inflated cardiovascular risk. If they ever experience bleeding gums, it wouldn't be a bad idea to have them screened using an oral or salivary DNA test.

Once again, the purpose of this book is not to reinforce things you are probably already doing – but to suggest a FEW things you could change which could make an enormous difference. It is also important to recognize the inherent weaknesses of continuing to offer only those tests that are part of the *lowest* 'Standard of Care'.

BIO TOOLS FOR MONITORING DISEASE – WELLNESS VIP

When I sit down with a physician I have some sense that they have already been testing or screening their patients. I don't know any physicians that don't do at least some testing as part of the workup for each patient's annual exam. In most cases they have been testing to diagnose risk factors for disease, they have used the test results as a metric to determine the existence and extent of cardiometabolic risk. In many cases, there has been limited action or sensitivity towards ongoing monitoring within a calendar year to drive to a specific therapeutic goal beyond risk management. In short, many physicians treat risk factors, not disease.

This is the case of many other industries where desired behavior is limited because the necessary tools to affect change in behavior just don't exist. Often, this has limited providers' abilities to go beyond simple risk assessment. Indeed – the standard of care is built around the concept of risk assessment – it doesn't really address treatment or management of disease nor therapeutic outcomes for patients. This rather parochial view of evaluating what is going on with the patient today then moving towards managing their risk factors, falls significantly short of a true wellness management plan. Managing disease by diagnosing, treating, monitoring, and making therapeutic recommendations and then reassessing the ongoing effect of those therapeutic recommendations is a tall order. Let's face it, 3rd party payers are also reticent to pay for anything but the basic standard of care. Optimal care remains an elusive dream in the minds of many health care providers.

When introducing this concept to a physician friend, a rather provocative way we have used to open the topic for discussion is to ask them about the most recent batch of tests they ran on a patient (either imaging or bio). Then we ask them why they ordered those specific tests. In other words, what are those tests going to reveal to get the patient to the ultimate goals of better therapeutic response and better health outcomes?

Many providers don't have a response to this question, or they may say the reason to test is a combination of A) it's a requirement to comply with the standard of care, or B) to address a specific patient complaint. Very few providers have the luxury to give much thought to the long-term goals of therapeutic response and better outcomes.

For many providers in the US, the primary objective is to manage the outcome of a lower LDL, or the improvement of blood glucose, blood pressure, or a very specific risk factor. The hope is that if we manage the risk factors, that will eventually improve the health outcomes.

That construct is based on public health directives which, of course, come from population health studies. Unfortunately, that may or may not work for the patient who is standing in front of you.

The reality is that heart attacks and strokes are still responsible for a full one third of the deaths in the US – and, unless we change our approach from managing risk factors to managing outcomes, that may not improve much more.

Overall patient outcome improvement seems too much of a stretch for many of the providers we speak to. Part of that reservation stems from the lack of tools to effectively and efficiently manage outcomes.

We believe that the Wellness VIP is a program, that once implemented, will bridge the gap from management of specific risk profiles, to the management of patient outcomes and that will ultimately lead to improved wellness. Of course, explicit in this belief is the concept that better wellness will result in patient's improved outlook on life, their improved mental health, improved interpersonal and familial relationships, improved sexual function and libido, more energy, and most importantly . . . increased quality and quantity of life. While this may seem like a tall order, let's break it down to the most important elements.

If we can reduce cardiovascular risk – and mortality, and this is a function of improved risk and lifestyle management, the patients may get to their ideal weight, they will eat healthier and eliminate poor health decisions like smoking or excessive sugar consumption. These lifestyle changes will naturally result in more energy, which could lead to improved exercise and metabolic changes which would improve vascular function.

The point is that small changes result in enormous benefits on the patient side. Unfortunately, many providers don't have the time to sell the benefits of improved outcomes because the system has forced them to see so many patients. Also, physicians are already discussing the importance of physical activity and risk management with the hope that these longer-term benefits will be realized. But the current discussions are hampered by the lack of efficient tools to connect the dots. By the time most physicians discuss whatever the patient came in to discuss, there is precious little time to dive into things like long range health goals and wellness.

The Wellness VIP portal enhances the communication between provider, the provider's office staff, and the patient, so that much of the needed messaging a provider does in the limited time during the office visit can be emphasized automatically via the use of technology and automation

In the Wellness VIP program, the patient has multiple interaction points as they utilize the portal to access their individualized health information. The program provides a natural focal point of communication and goal-driven behavior that can easily guide future visits to a common rationale and goal centered health outcome.

Some years ago, we spent a considerable amount of time and money to put together this tool that would bind together patients and their providers. Recently, rules have forced medical practices to implement Electronic Medical Records (EMR) systems where they can track each patient's medical history and treatment plan. This information is often stored outside the purview of patients, in fact, it can be quite cumbersome to print out even the most basic pieces of information which physicians want to share with their patients.

Subsequent to many of these conversations I partnered with the former President of Berkeley HeartLab, Frank Ruderman, to create a solution that would resonate with both physicians and patients.

You may remember that Berkeley HeartLab single handedly changed the face of health care by introducing advanced lipid panels, including lipid fractionation and genetic testing to better inform physicians and patients about the nature of their disease and the efficacy of their treatment recommendations. Berkeley was very successful at creating treatment centers that advanced a more holistic approach to cardiovascular care, by integrating the elements of BHL test results, diet, exercise, and medicines.

This business grew exponentially from just over a $1MM each year in revenue, to nearly $100MM per year. It was eventually sold to Celera for $195MM. Frank was the architect of this direction and was hugely successful, along with his dedicated employees, at creating a change in the landscape of healthcare and cardiovascular wellness management.

Our original concept was to take what Berkeley had created and advance it to the next level of services that Berkeley was never able to achieve. The outcrop of that endeavor was a new company: Wellness VIP where the VIP stands for Vascular Improvement Program, and, of course, where the primary focus is on Wellness.

Embedded in the Wellness VIP platform are essentially three separate portals: one portal designed specifically for physicians, one for coaches and other administrative staff in the provider's office, and one for patients. We affectionately called this tool our Electronic Medical Communication System (EMCS), a stark contrast to the Electronic Medical Record (EMR) systems which merely host patient medical records.

The EMCS not only hosts the patient's medical records, but it also facilitates the communication of test results, therapeutic recommendations, and a comprehensive action plan designed to help each patient achieve specific wellness outcomes. Since it is highly unlikely you have been introduced to this tool, I have included a few screen shots from the Physicians and Patient portals to help highlight some of the features.

One of the things that should surprise you is that this program is free to the providers and patients using it. That is right – there is no cost to the physician or the patient. The program is monetized through agreements with the blood laboratories who process the samples. This was a crucial element of the program. Please keep this in mind as you review the features of this powerful and effective program.

WELLNESS VIP - PROVIDER PORTAL

The EMCS is a system that allows the physician and their staff to communicate directly with patients regarding health history and medical directives, including prescriptive information. This is a dynamic interaction between the provider and their patients that facilitates a personalized approach to understanding and characterizing preexisting risk. For those who subscribe to Medicare and Medicaid, this system also helps with compliance on the quality systems and reporting required by MIPS or MACRS.

Each one of the patients that is part of the Wellness VIP program is introduced to it because they had been pre-determined to have some type of cardio-metabolic or inflammatory vascular risk, which was characterized in prior clinical visits with specific ICD-10 codes. These patients now come to the Wellness VIP program to get a better and more integrated understanding of their risks, to further characterize it, and ultimately to get a personalized treatment program that they can follow. The program allows the provider to then follow and iteratively monitor progression of patient wellness over time, in order to achieve the therapeutic objectives and improved outcomes.

The purpose of the first visit, or what we call the baseline determination for ongoing monitoring, is to take a look at a comprehensive set of tests which are organized into five pillars, categories, or verticals: 1) *Cardiovascular and Pre-Diabetes;* 2) *Thyroid*; 3) *Inflammation* and an entire set of Physical Diagnostic Tests (CIMT, Endothelial Function, etc.); 4) a set of 'Wellness Plus' analytes including *Hormone Balance;* and then 5) a therapeutic response monitoring set which includes *Pharmacogenomics* and if needed, *Micro Nutrient Testing (MNT)*. All of these panels are designed to help personalize the patient's medical treatment plans.

The purpose of the provider site is to utilize a comprehensive set of analytes to characterize the existing risk of the patient and then to integrate those analytes into an approach that will give the physician a recommendation to affect a set of therapeutic responses or outcomes. Behind the scenes in the portal is a series of algorithms which are created based on the most current literature. These algorithmic rules take the unique combinations of results from each patient's testing and then prescribes a recommended set of treatment considerations. These recommendations include Diet, Exercise, and other Lifestyle recommendations, along with any pharmaceutical considerations.

The portal stops short of making dose or brand choices, leaving those final decisions to the provider. The provider can add to or remove any of the algorithmic recommendations before finalizing the plan. The provider then takes these recommendations and chooses which ones he/she sees as relevant to the patient. Once the desired therapeutic response has been selected, the provider approves the treatment plan and makes it a part of each patient's treatment goals.

These goals are then communicated to the patient and, following a final approval by the physician, the plan appears in the patient's individual portal for their review and implementation.

In the Physician Portal landing page below (Figure 5) you can see the following labeled information:

1 – Basic demographic information which identifies the patient and basic information about their health.

2 – The most recent displayed testing history.

3 - Pull-down menus which allow instant access to any historical testing results conducted within the program.

4 – The algorithmically assigned Risk Summary which is accompanied by editable Treatment Considerations. The Treatment Considerations outline a suggested or recommended intervention which also can be edited.

5 – Results are displayed with traditional Green, Yellow, and Red-light indicators to quickly characterize the patient's test results.

Additional display options are available by selecting Tabular or Graphical view (Figure 7). These display options offer clarity when comparing current to previous results.

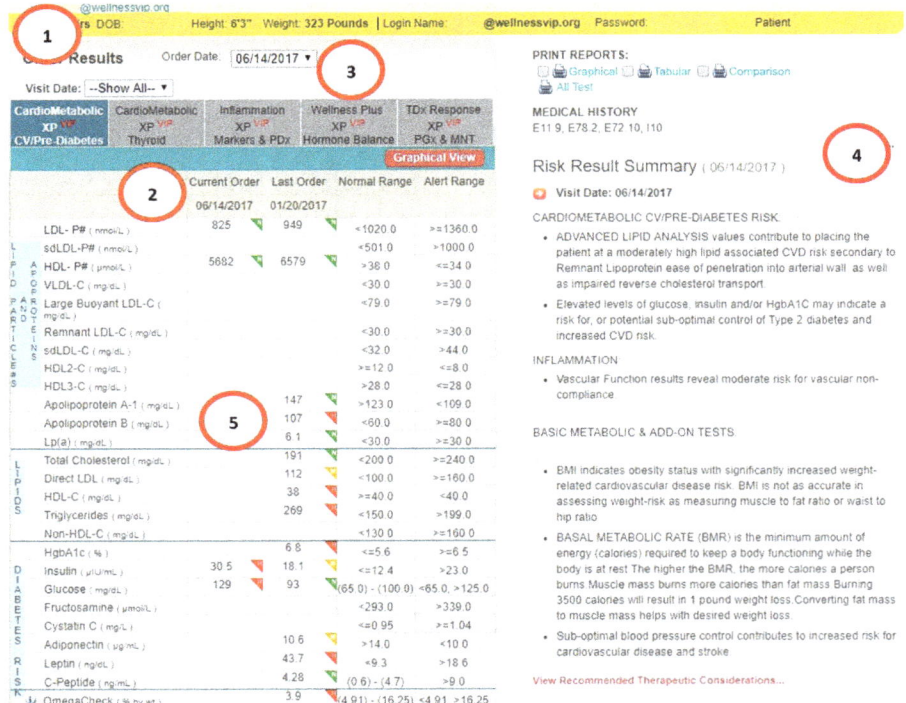

Figure 5

If needed, the provider can search the Order History and see a larger range of testing date results which helps to tell a story (Figure 6). This is particularly useful when the patient is making significant improvements and is compliant – but also when the opposite is true. Imagine the effect this data could have on a non-compliant patient whose results were getting worse on every visit. Over and over we have seen access to test results affect patients emotionally providing additional value as an effective compliance tool. The provider can also see any of the analyte results in a bar graph presentation that paints a clearer picture of each patient's progression of wellness. (Figure 7).

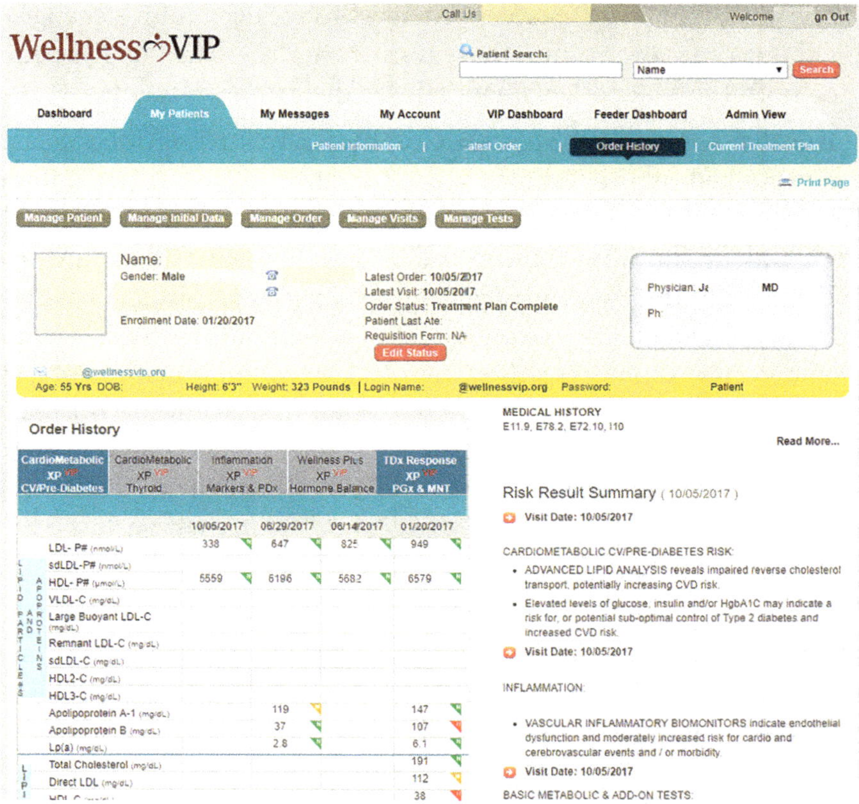

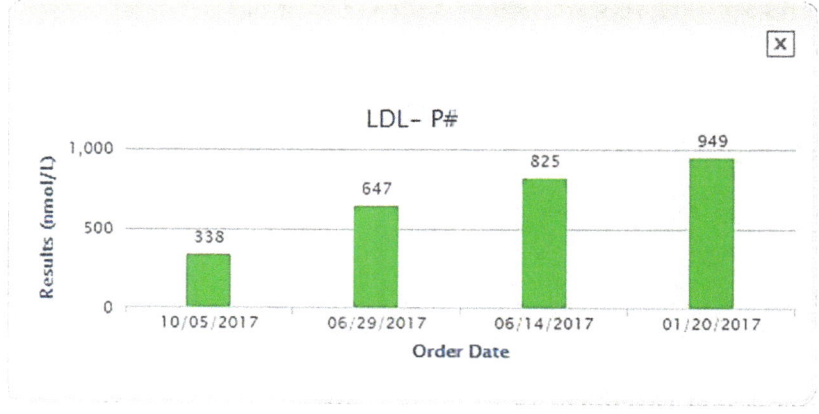

Figure 6

Figure 7

The physician portal enables providers to see even minor changes in patient outcomes over time. These results are also posted on the patient facing portal so that patients, too, can see their improvements.

Another viewing option is the Graphical / Tabular option. We have already looked at the Tabular view, but the Graphical presentation offers the additional benefit of helping patients and physicians to better understand how far into the Red, Yellow, or Green categories they may be in their wellness continuum. For example, the patient in (Figure 8) has an alert value on Direct LDL that puts them in a caution or Yellow zone. Looking at the graphical representation, however, we can see how close this patient is to a value that would be normal or Green. This information can be used to motivate patient compliance. By showing a patient how close they are to a normal result, we may be able to motivate them to make the necessary changes to push the value into the Green zone.

This view provides additional insight we don't necessarily get in a Tabular type report. Not all Red conditions are the same. The same could be said of Yellow and Green conditions. Understanding how far into each condition a patient appears in each of these fields is valuable insight not available in traditional result reports which are typically reported in a Tabular format. Note in the example below (Figure 8) that this patient's LDL-P particle number is barely over the border for Green. This may indicate the need for additional caution. By contrast, the same patient's Lp(a) results are well into the Green area.

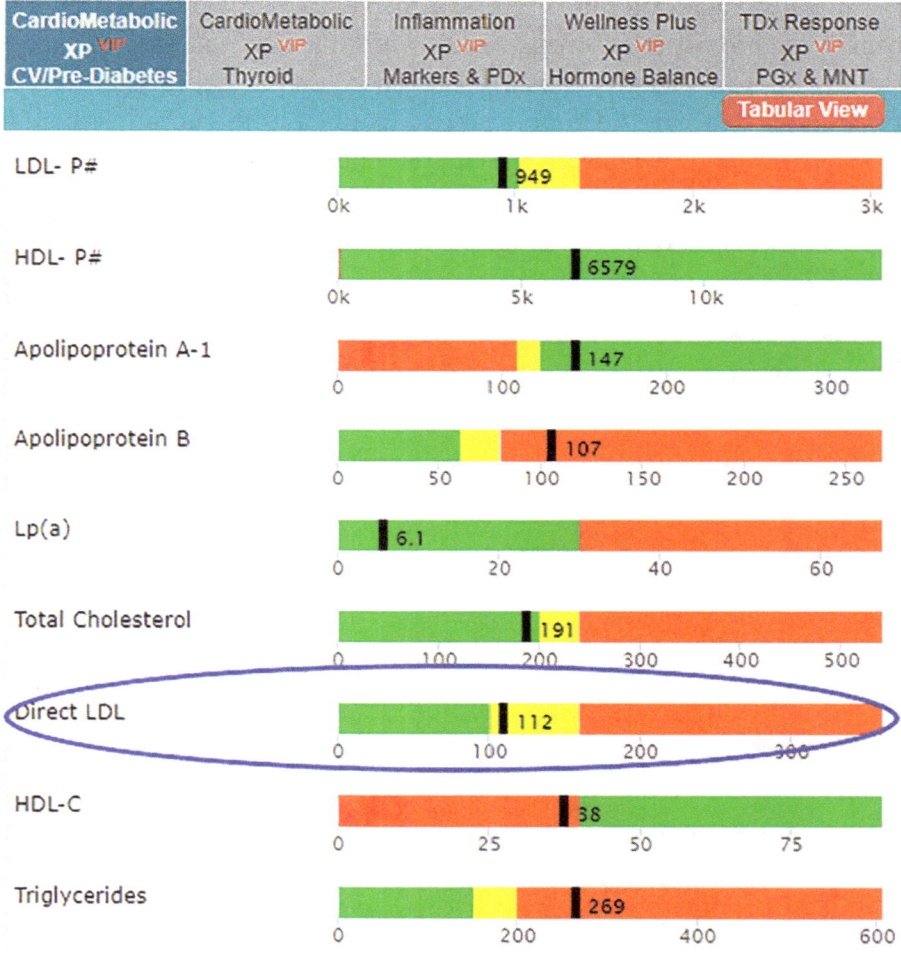

CardioMetabolic XP VIP CV/Pre-Diabetes	CardioMetabolic XP VIP Thyroid	Inflammation XP VIP Markers & PDx	Wellness Plus XP VIP Hormone Balance	TDx Response XP VIP PGx & MNT

Tabular View

LDL- P# — 949 (0k, 1k, 2k, 3k)

HDL- P# — 6579 (0k, 5k, 10k)

Apolipoprotein A-1 — 147 (0, 100, 200, 300)

Apolipoprotein B — 107 (0, 50, 100, 150, 200, 250)

Lp(a) — 6.1 (0, 20, 40, 60)

Total Cholesterol — 191 (0, 100, 200, 300, 400, 500)

Direct LDL — 112 (0, 100, 200, 300)

HDL-C — 38 (0, 25, 50, 75)

Triglycerides — 269 (0, 200, 400, 600)

Figure 8

The integrated reporting allows the provider to make decisions about the urgency of care and the aggressiveness of the therapeutic intervention. By monitoring the patient's results over time, providers can also see the effect of the intervention to see if it has been efficacious or conversely, if it needs to be escalated.

In most cases, monitoring 2 -3 times each year provides adequate oversight into whether treatment is working and whether a change should be considered regarding the dose, the drug, or the lifestyle parameters that have been prescribed. In all cases the portal is there to help physicians drive toward the desired outcomes.

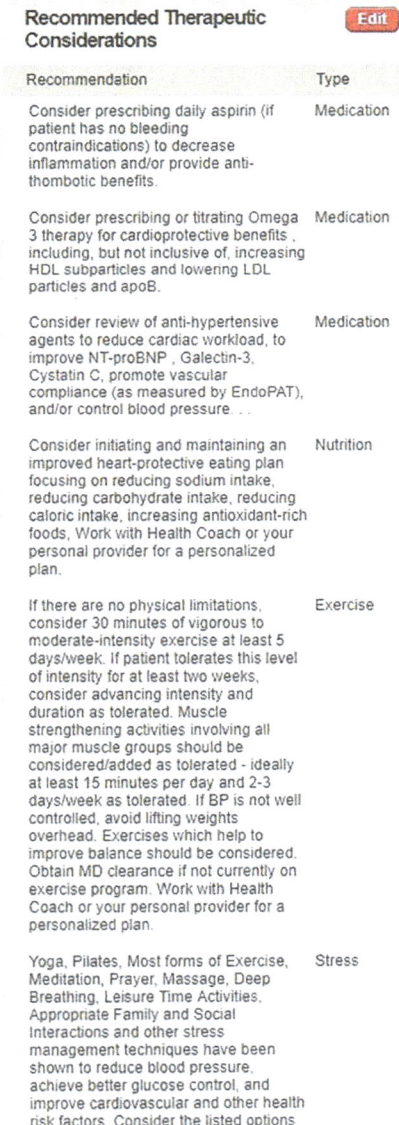

Figure 9

It's important to note that both the Risk Results Summaries, the Therapeutic Considerations, and the Goals are set to populate automatically based on the algorithms governing each analyte's result conditions. Having said that, it is also important to note that all these can be edited before submitting to a patient so that the patient sees only what the physician feels is prudent. The exception is the testing results themselves, of course.

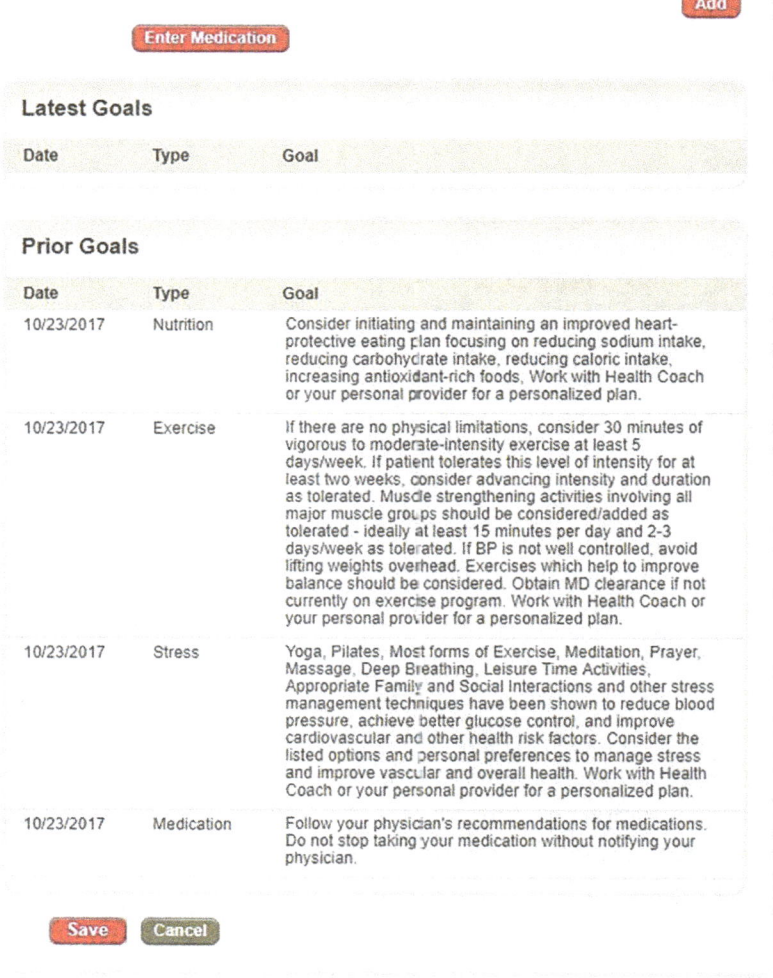

Figure 10

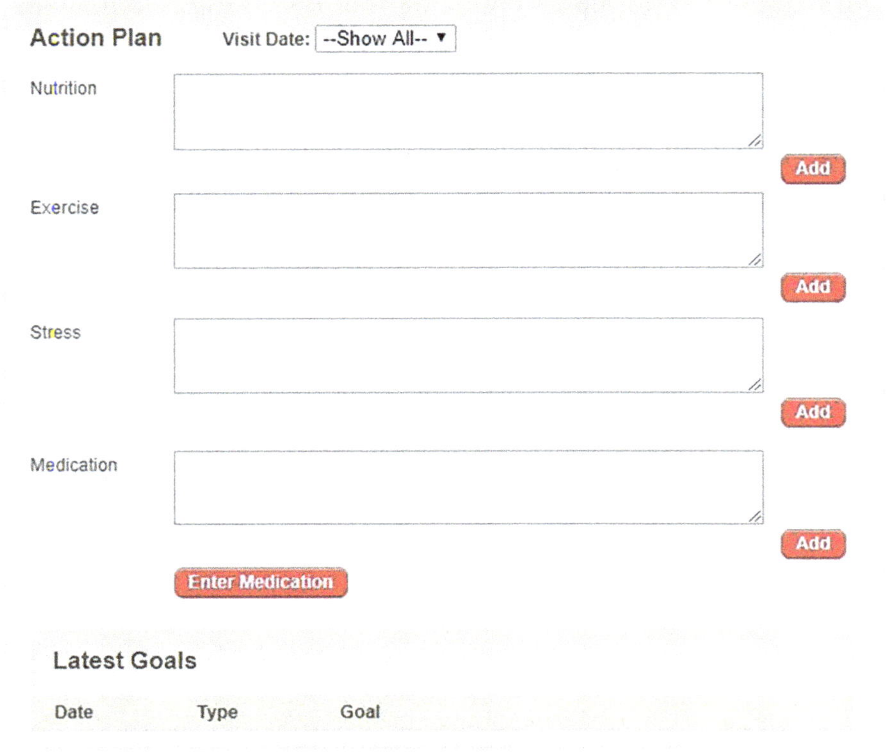

Action Plan   Visit Date: --Show All-- ▼

Nutrition

[Add]

Exercise

[Add]

Stress

[Add]

Medication

[Add]

[Enter Medication]

Latest Goals

Date	Type	Goal

Image 11

This entire data set of test Results, Risk Summaries, Therapeutic Considerations, Action Plans, and Prior Goals sits on an AWS (Amazon) cloud server in an extremely secure and encrypted environment where it is maintained in perpetuity. This repository of data is always available much like any cloud based system, so that every time a patient comes back in for an appointment, the Medical Assistants or front office staff can bring that patient's information up for review and action.

This integrated approach of test results, driven through algorithmic Results Summary then to a detailed Therapeutic Treatment Considerations allows the provider to develop an action plan where the prior goals become a permanent part of each patient record along with the goals that the patient sets for themselves on their own portal. The integrated approach drives better patient compliance through ongoing monitoring and reporting which ultimately drives better outcomes.

Finally, the Print Report function allows the provider to decide what information is printed for a patient, and how it is presented (e.g. Tabular or Graphical presentation). The provider can choose to compare results, or to print specific pieces of information. Since the MIPS and MACRS quality programs require a printed plan, this too is available for print from both the Physician's portal and the Coaching portals. (Figure 12). Implicit in the Print function is the ability to print PDF's sent from the various laboratories who provide results. The portal can import reports from any company who provides their results to Wellness VIP in a PDF or HL7 compliant upload, or in a hard copy format which can be scanned and entered into the system.

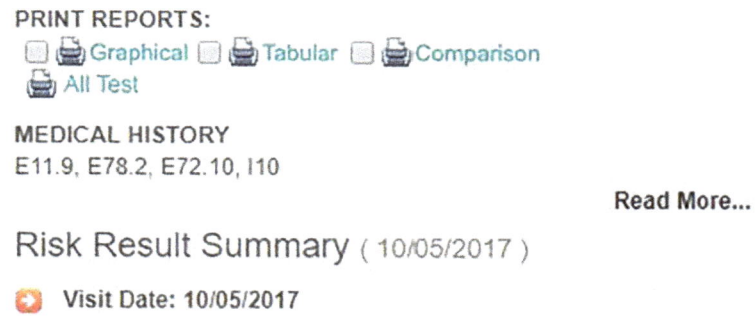

Figure 12

WELLNESS VIP - Patient Portal

The Patient Portal features the Action Plan and Goals agreed to by the provider and selected for communication. This will always include the patient's own risk result reports from the various laboratories. Every recommendation that the provider has made and that they want the patient to see is accessible and visualized via the Patient Portal (Image 13). The initial landing page provides quick access to the patient's health overview to include Height, Weight, Blood Pressure, etc. These criteria can be modified by the patient which is useful for at-home monitoring of key metrics.

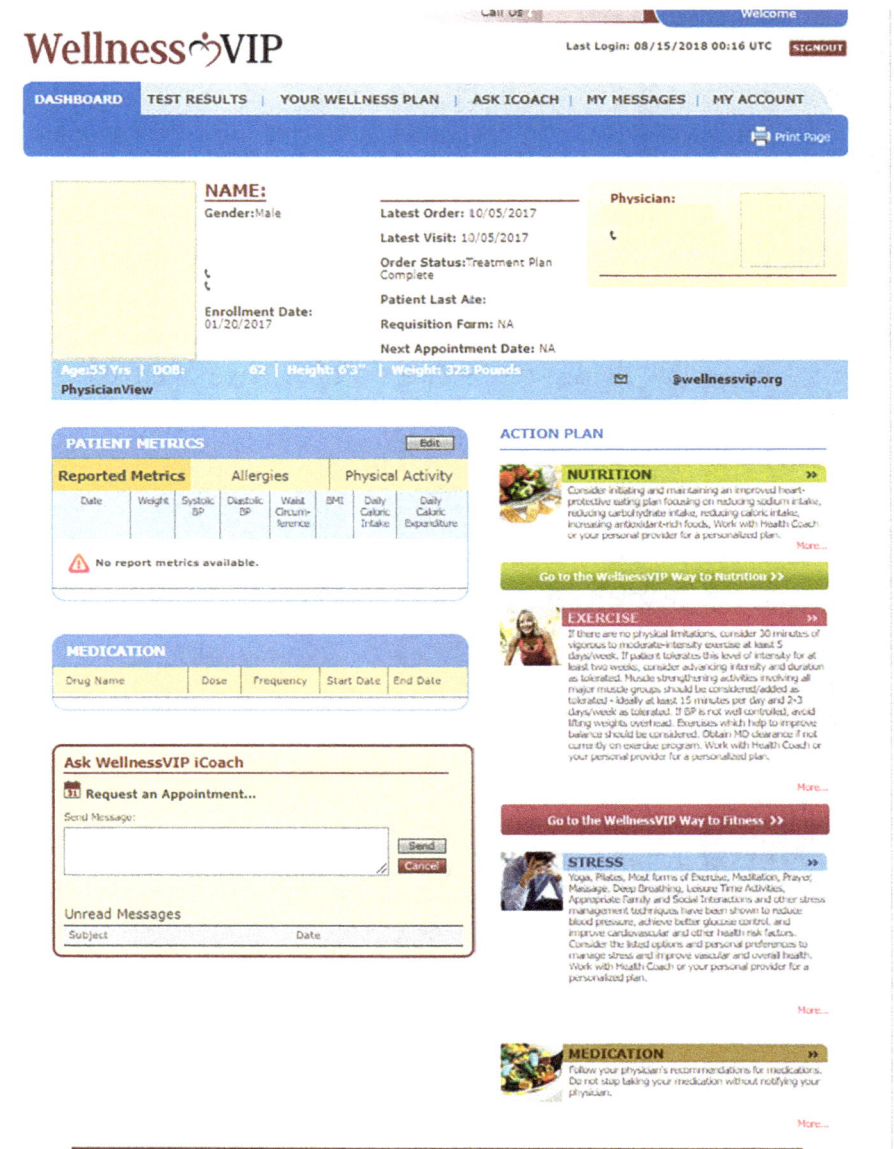

Image 13

Of course, the information is organized in a user friendly format which is more readily accomplished in the context of a webpage. Instead of just presenting test results in a manner that will be consumed by the patient without understanding or context, the patient portal organizes the data along with the Action Plan as prescribed and directed by the provider. This information is combined with specific Goals which drive towards a mutually agreed upon improved wellness outcome.

Each specific goal can be accessed in the extended view which expands into a more clearly defined and patient friendly view of the recommendations (Image 14). The ultimate objective is to give each patient a personalized Action Plan which they can follow. This Action Plan is driven by all the test metrics which have been completed, analyzed, and integrated for them by their provider.

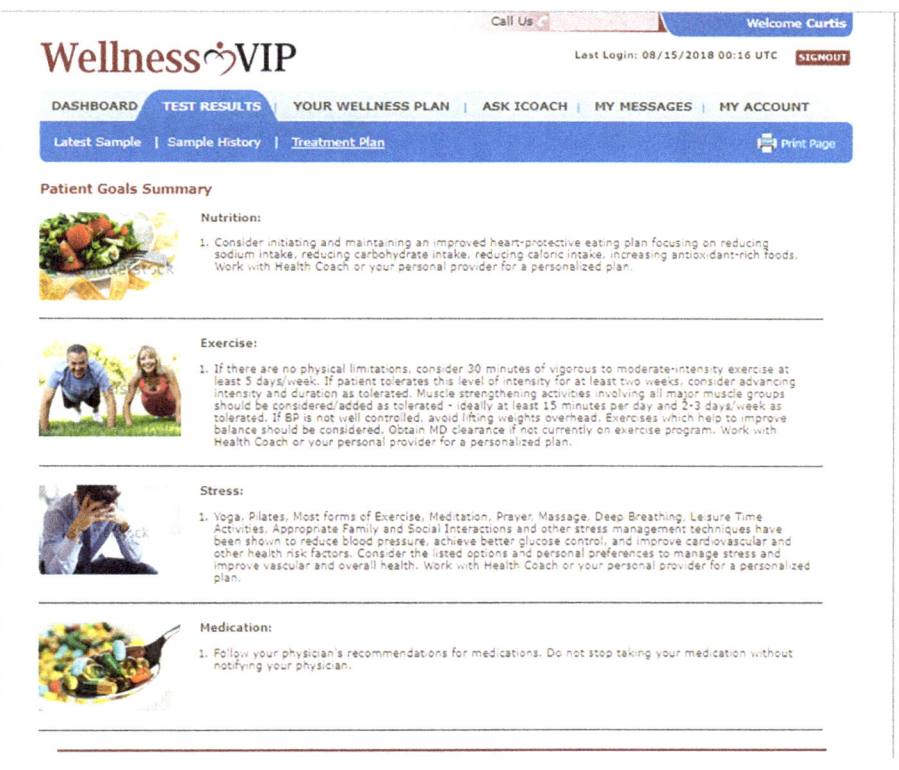

Image 14

When our patient, Curtis, clicks on his test results (Image 15), he can then see his test results which are on the cloud and he can refer back to them at any point from virtually any computer. This keeps the results top of mind because access and reminders about the mutually agreed upon plan is always there. Once again, Curtis can see his individual Sample History (Image 15).

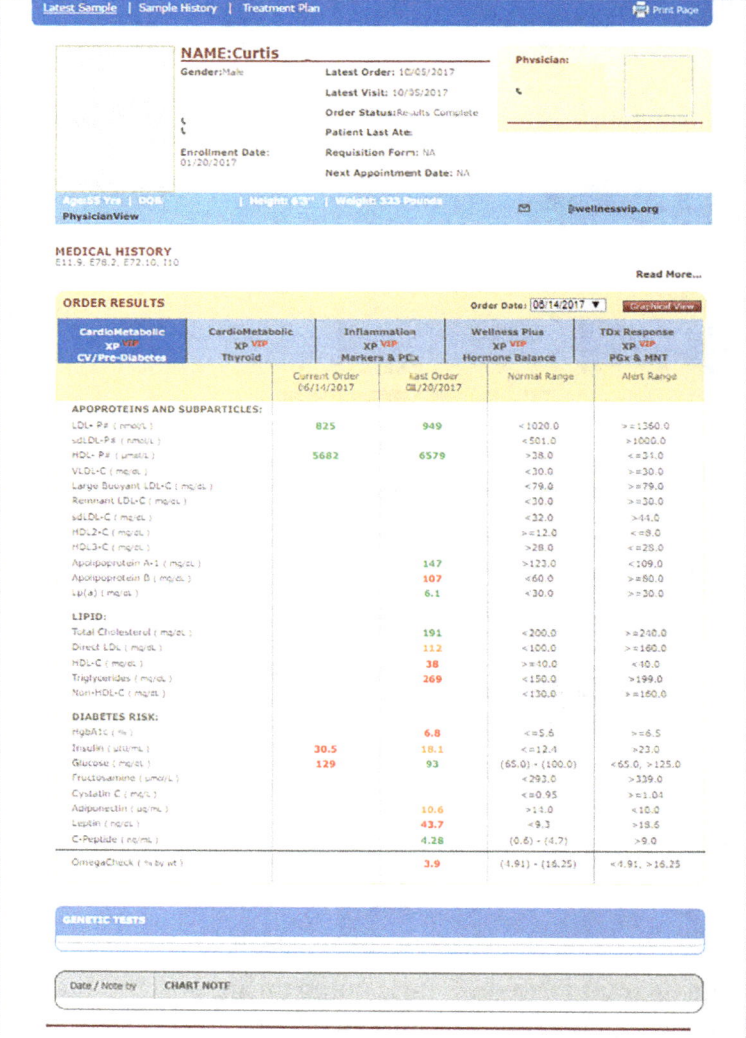

Image 15

Should Curtis desire to see his results in the Graphical format, that option is easily accessible with the touch of a button (Image 16).

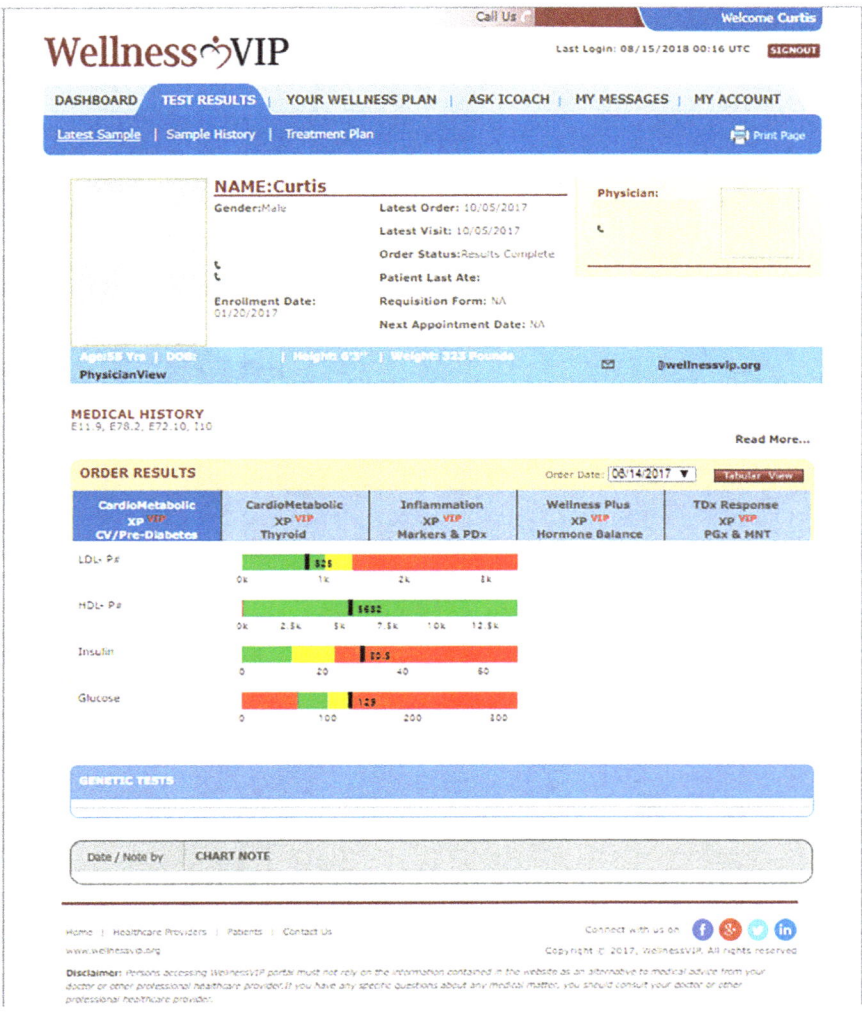

Image 16

Should he want to see how he is doing on any specific analyte, he can drill down on that specific test. This enables him to track his progression in the same way the provider does to underscore improvement or the lack thereof. (Image 17)

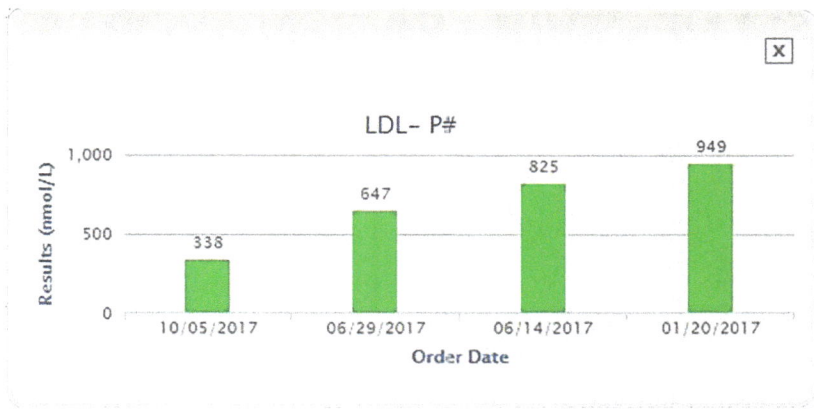

Image 17

The purpose of the Patient Portal is not to develop the personalized treatment plan, but instead to take the prescribed personalized treatment plan, to understand it, and then be guided by what is prescribed on the portal (in concert with the provider) to better implement the plan. The entire purpose of the integrated Action Plan is to direct that behavior or behaviors which will assist the patient in achieving the desired therapeutic objective for his improved outcomes.

Although the objectives are different in each of these portals, they have much of the same content. However, it's important to note that the Patient Portal does not have any of the algorithms, or Risk Summaries, or the Recommended Treatment Considerations. Instead, the Patient Portal has the most current recommended Action Plan which was derived, at least in part, from that content.

In short, the patient does not have anything in the way of individualized treatment content which directs him except that which was specifically released to him by his provider. So the conclusion reached by the provider from the other data in the Physician's portal is what is ultimately presented to each patient in the Patient portal.

WELLNESS VIP - PATIENT PORTAL HEALTHY LIVING CONTENT

In addition to the individualized health plan which is directed by the provider, the Wellness VIP Patient portal is loaded with content designed to help each individual live a healthier life. This content is accessible from the top menu and is broken into four categories: *Nutrition, Exercise, Stress,* and *Medication*. We will explore some of these submenus below.

NUTRITION

The Nutrition section of the Patient portal is designed to provide content relating to more healthy food choices. This Nutrition related content includes calorie and portion control, a food diary, and food group variety insight (Image 18, Image 18a).

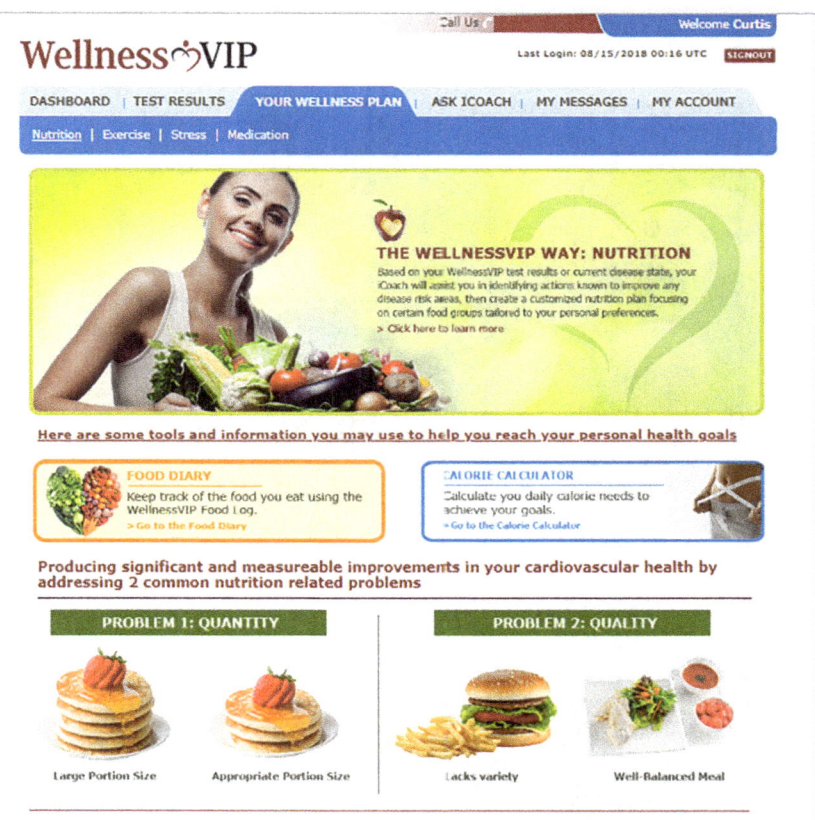

Image 18

SOLUTION 1: PORTION CONTROL

Notice the 2 plates below – you are able to cut 500 calories from the plate at the bottom by changing how much you eat of different foods

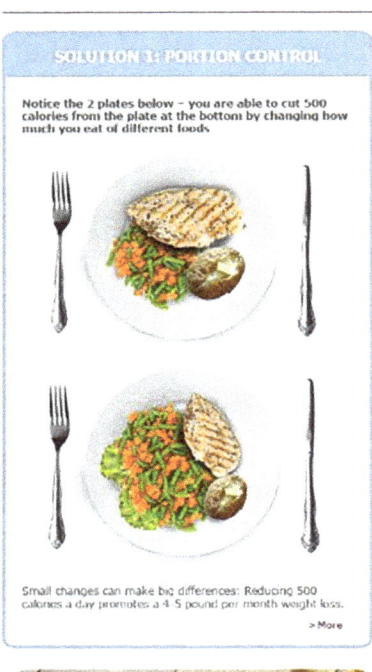

Small changes can make big differences: Reducing 500 calories a day promotes a 4-5 pound per month weight loss.

> More

SOLUTION 2: FOOD GROUP VARIETY

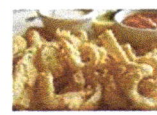

Does this plate look familiar? Unfortunately, a typical diet promotes development of cardiovascular disease through foods high in calories, saturated fat, sodium, refined sugar and low quantities of vitamins, minerals and fiber.

By changing the type of foods that you eat, you can reduce your consumption of fats and sugars. Click on the diagram below to learn how eating certain foods can help decrease cardiovascular disease risk by by reducing inflammation or plaque development, improving cholesterol levels, controlling diabetes, managing hypertension and improving metabolism.

> Click on the wheel below to learn more.

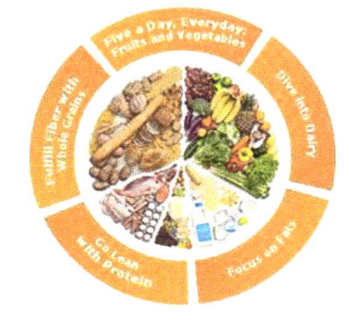

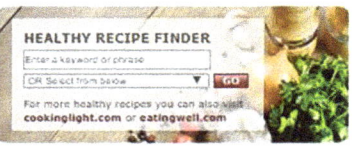

HEALTHY RECIPE FINDER

Enter a keyword or phrase

OR Select from below ▼ | GO |

For more healthy recipes you can also visit cookinglight.com or eatingwell.com

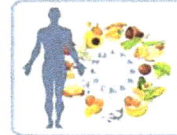

ALL ABOUT MICRONUTRIENTS

WellnessVIP partners with SpectraCell in offering micronutrient testing. Micronutrient testing can test for nutrients that promote good health.

> Go to Micronutrient Testing

|O| HEALTHY EATING TIPS

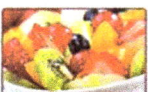

Adding more fruits and Vegetables

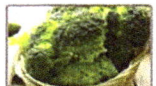

Healthy Bites

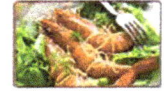

Dining out tips

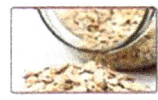

Fiber foods

> Click here for more HEALTHY EATING TIPS

♥ LEARN, SHARE, GET EXPERT VIEWS

Image 18a

The Patient portal also provides useful links to nationally recognized thought leaders and organizations who provide valuable health insights. (Image 19)

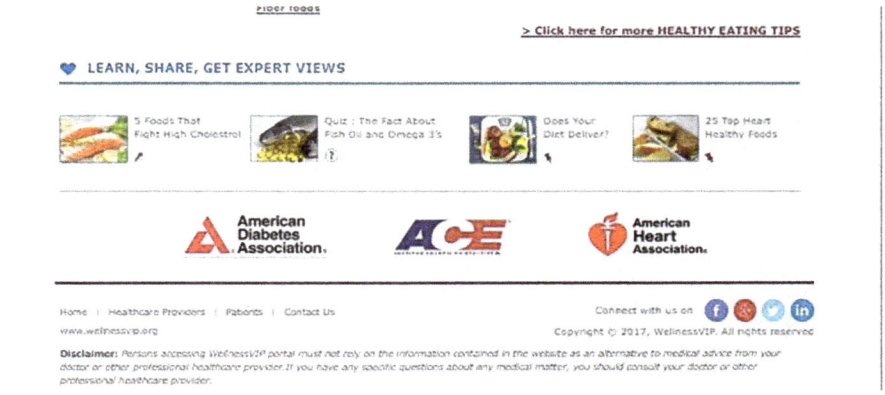

Image 19

The calorie counter provides detailed metabolic advice based on each patient's individualized metabolic profile. (Image 20)

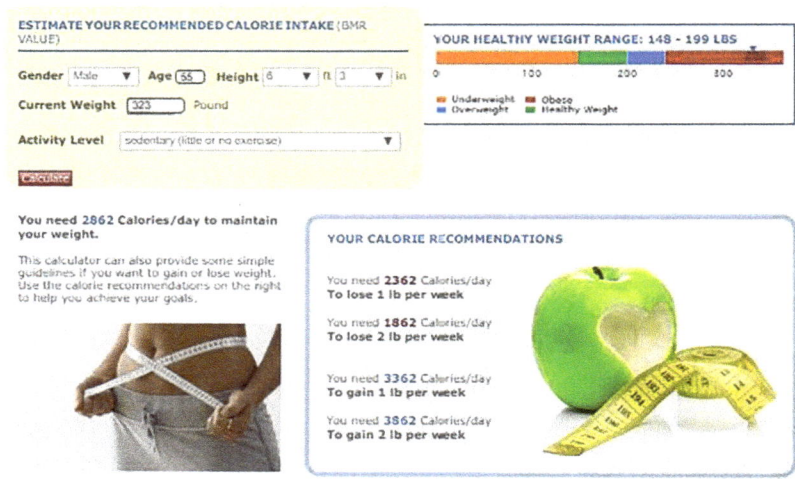

Image 20

One of the first steps in helping people make better lifestyle choices is helping them to identify and track their health habits. Eating is one of the most important of those habits. The Food Diary provides a location for patients to keep an active diary of their daily food consumption. This feature includes a comprehensive menu of food choices, including a list of foods from the most popular fast food restaurants. The obvious purpose of this diary is to facilitate the tracking of caloric intake with the goal of identifying opportunities for improvement in this area (Image 21).

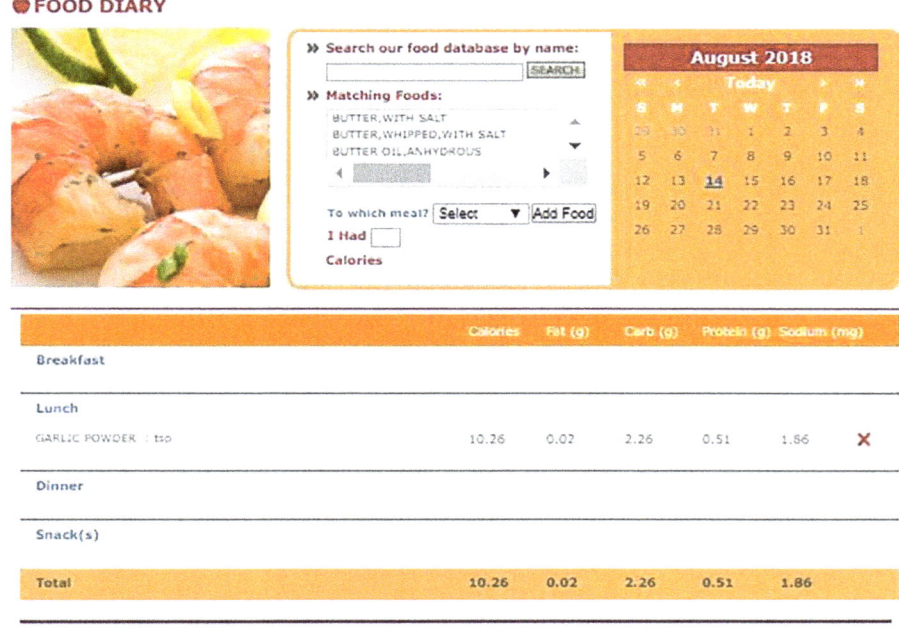

Image 21

Another aspect of eating and diet control is learning about appropriate portion size. Many patients struggle to know how much they should be eating. Diet books are full of verbiage about the number of ounces of protein or vegetables. Many patients couldn't tell you easily what a 6 oz portion of protein looks like. The Patient portal helps address these concerns in a visually easy to understand format (Image 22).

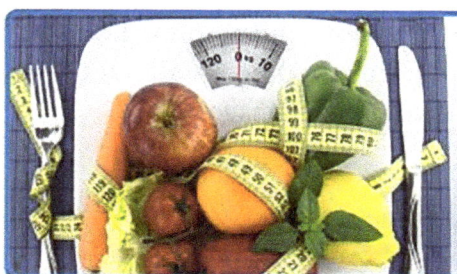

HOW THE WELLNESS VIP PORTION CONTROL PLAN REDUCES YOUR HEART RISK

Your iCoach will work with you to understand your current diet habits and provide guidance on proper portion control

WHY IS PORTION CONTROL IMPORTANT?

Portion control is a critical part of successful weight loss and weight management. The WellnessVIP Portion Size Plate gives you easy-to-understand guidelines to help you avoid some common portion-size pitfalls. Portions can be controlled in 3 ways:
1. Managing what you eat when
2. Controlling how much you eat
3. Monitoring calorie intake

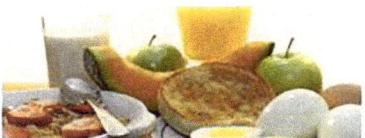

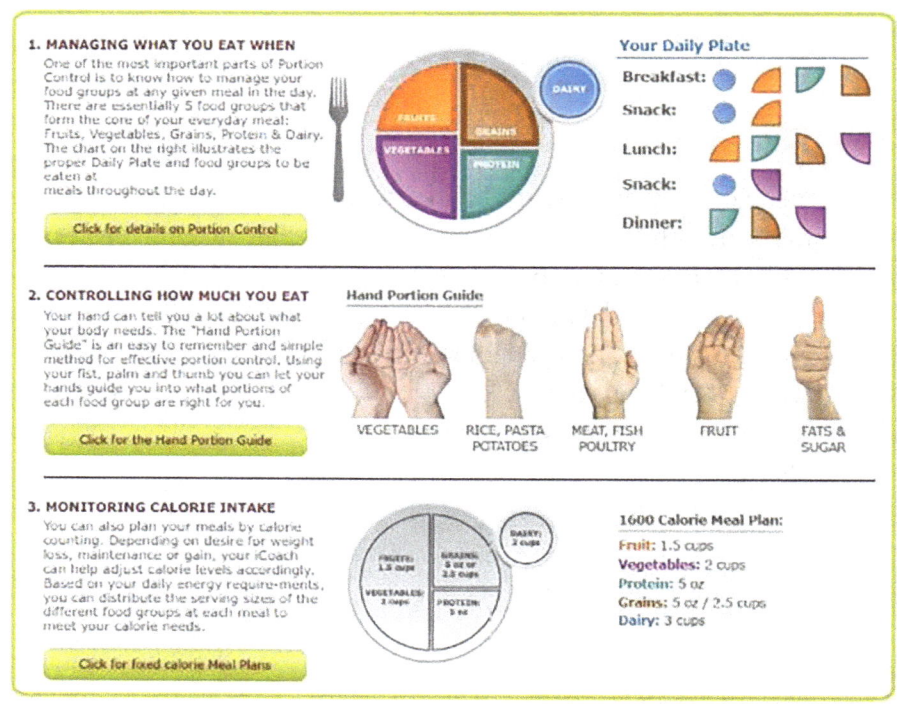

Image 22

A healthy recipe finder is provided for motivated patients who may need assistance changing the way they prepare food and the ingredients they put into their food. The simple pull-down menu provides instant access to a plethora of recipe choices and links to other useful sites which can assist them in improving their food choices (Image 23).

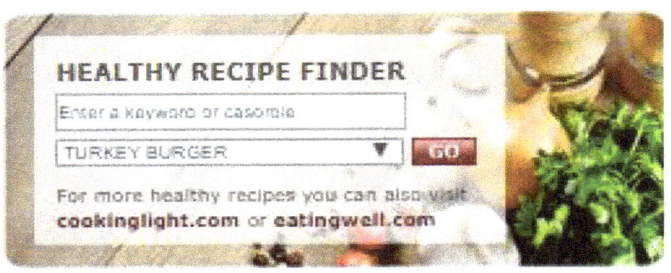

Image 23

MICRONUTRIENTS

For some patients, particularly those with specific vitamin, mineral, antioxidant, or other Micro Nutrient deficiencies, getting to an ideal weight or body mass might be particularly difficult. These patients tend to lack the energy and vitality many healthy people take for granted. Micro Nutrient testing is available though the Wellness VIP program. The Patient portal provides a thorough and detailed explanation of what each of these nutrients mean and how they can affect good health. (Image 24, Image 25)

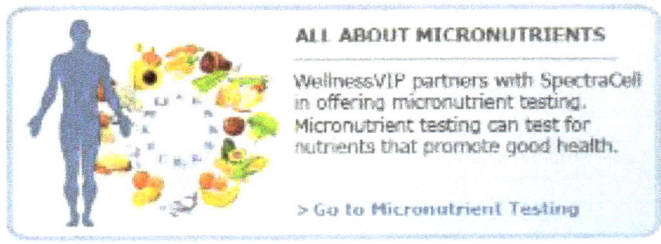

Image 24

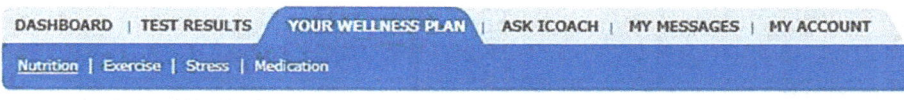

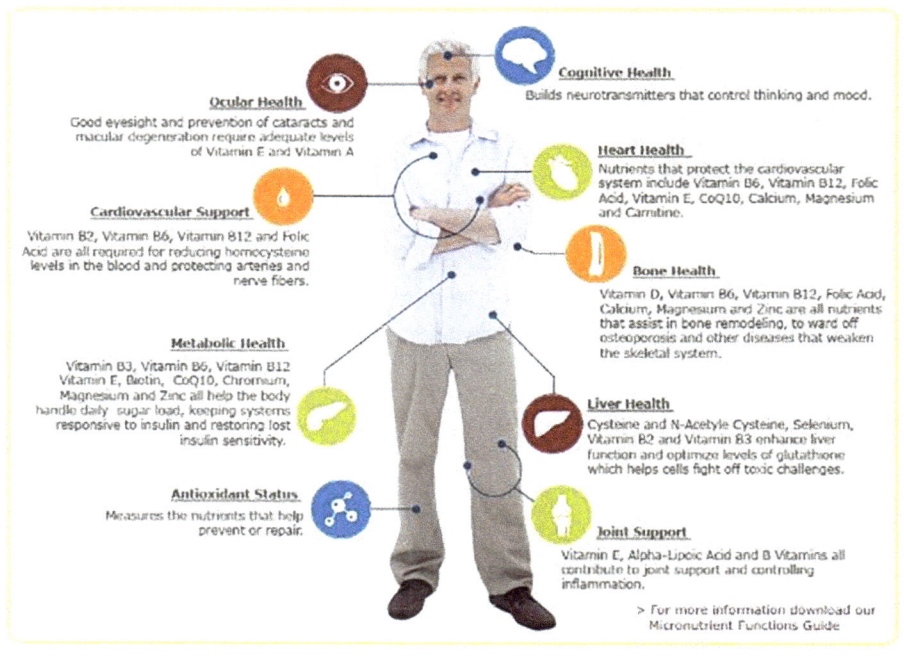

Image 25

A deeper dive into five specific nutrient profiles reveals the unique combinations of Micro Nutrients and how they affect each of these desired outcomes. The five specific wellness health profiles may relate directly to the specific or desired outcome agreed to by both provider and patient. The five outcome specific profiles which are addressed through the Micro Nutrients section of the Patient Portal include: ***Decrease Inflammation & Plaque Formation, Improve Cholesterol & Lipids, Prevent and/or Control Diabetes, Manage Hypertension,*** and ***Improve***

Metabolic Status. Each of these is addressed via graphic wheels which address the various nutrients involved in the desired health outcome (Image 26).

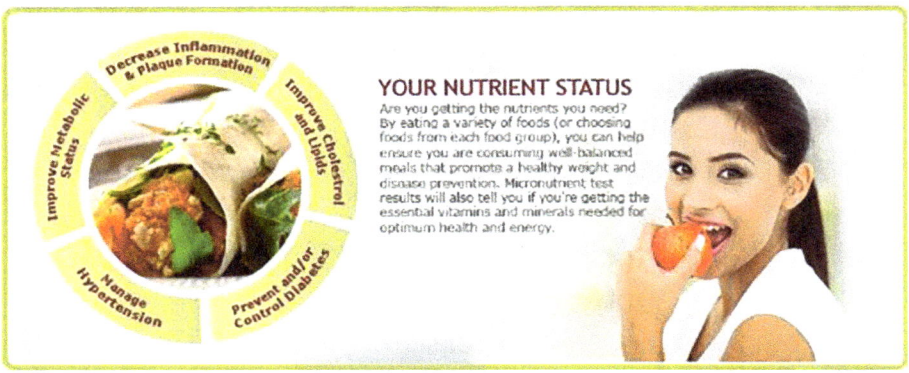

YOUR NUTRIENT STATUS

Are you getting the nutrients you need? By eating a variety of foods (or choosing foods from each food group), you can help ensure you are consuming well-balanced meals that promote a healthy weight and disease prevention. Micronutrient test results will also tell you if you're getting the essential vitamins and minerals needed for optimum health and energy.

Click on the categories in the circle above or the table below to learn how Micronutrient Testing provides information influencing each of the five cardiovascular disease risk areas.

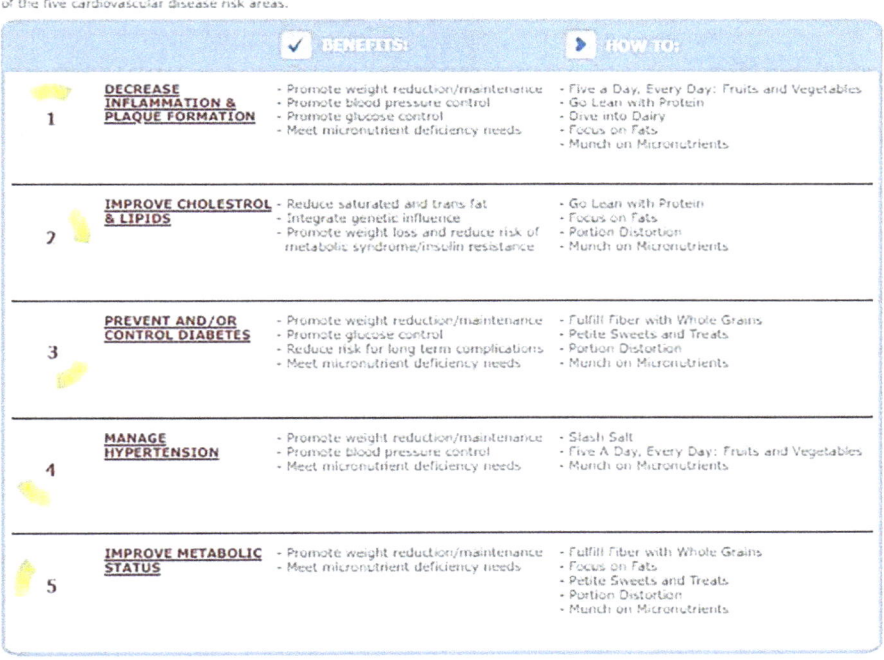

		✔ BENEFITS:	▶ HOW TO:
1	**DECREASE INFLAMMATION & PLAQUE FORMATION**	- Promote weight reduction/maintenance - Promote blood pressure control - Promote glucose control - Meet micronutrient deficiency needs	- Five a Day, Every Day: Fruits and Vegetables - Go Lean with Protein - Dive into Dairy - Focus on Fats - Munch on Micronutrients
2	**IMPROVE CHOLESTROL & LIPIDS**	- Reduce saturated and trans fat - Integrate genetic influence - Promote weight loss and reduce risk of metabolic syndrome/insulin resistance	- Go Lean with Protein - Focus on Fats - Portion Distortion - Munch on Micronutrients
3	**PREVENT AND/OR CONTROL DIABETES**	- Promote weight reduction/maintenance - Promote glucose control - Reduce risk for long term complications - Meet micronutrient deficiency needs	- Fulfill Fiber with Whole Grains - Petite Sweets and Treats - Portion Distortion - Munch on Micronutrients
4	**MANAGE HYPERTENSION**	- Promote weight reduction/maintenance - Promote blood pressure control - Meet micronutrient deficiency needs	- Slash Salt - Five A Day, Every Day: Fruits and Vegetables - Munch on Micronutrients
5	**IMPROVE METABOLIC STATUS**	- Promote weight reduction/maintenance - Meet micronutrient deficiency needs	- Fulfill Fiber with Whole Grains - Focus on Fats - Petite Sweets and Treats - Portion Distortion - Munch on Micronutrients

Image 26

Inflammation and Plaque Formation (Image 27)

DECREASE INFLAMMATION & PLAQUE FORMATION

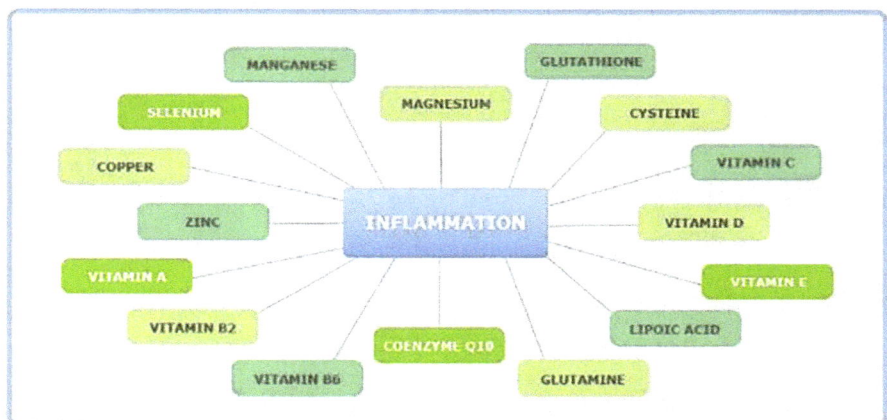

MANGANESE
Cofactor to the powerful antioxidant superoxide dismutase that fights inflammation within cells.

MAGNESIUM
Deficiency activates proinflammatory chemicals called cytokines; Deficiency will also kick start a damaging immune response by activating cells called leukocytes and macrophages.

GLUTATHIONE
Repairs damage to cells caused by inflammation; Regulates the production of pro-inflammatory cytokines; Recycles vitamins C and E.

CYSTEINE
Protects organs such as blood vessels, brain and liver from inflammatory damage; Precursor to glutathione production; Supplementation with Nacetyl cysteine raises glutathione.

VITAMIN C
Low vitamin C linked to inflammation; Inversely related to C-reactive protein (CRP), a marker for systemic inflammation; Increases glutathione.

VITAMIN D
Potent modulator of inflammation; Helps turn off chronic inflammatory responses; Inhibits pro-inflammatory cytokine production.

VITAMIN E
Limits destructive cell behavior caused by inflammatory enzymes gone wild; Reduces damage from tumor necrosis factor alpha (TNF-a); Deficiency predisposes a person to inflammationrelated diseases.

LIPOIC ACID
Neutralizes free radicals caused by uncontrolled inflammation in both water and lipid phases of the cell; Protects endothelial cells from inflammation; Regenerates other antioxidants such as vitamin E, C and glutathione.

GLUTAMINE
Decreases cytokine production; Invokes an anti-inflammatory response; Precursor to glutathione.

COENZYME Q10
Decreases several inflammatory markers (CRP and IL-6) in supplementation trials; Affects genes that control response to inflammatory stress.

VITAMIN B6
Low B6 status is linked to high levels of CRP and systemic inflammation.

VITAMIN B2
Riboflavin (B2) helps minimize pain associated with inflammation; Detoxifies homocysteine, an amino acid that indirectly causes inflammation in various tissues.

VITAMIN A
Regulates the cellular immune response to inflammatory signals; Deficiency increases the severity of chronic inflammation; Zinc depletion lowers vitamin A status.

ZINC
Inflammation raises demand for zinc; Pro-inflammatory chemicals (cytokines) dose dependently decrease in response to zinc repletion.

COPPER
Deficiency lowers enzyme activity (such as superoxide dismutase) that fights inflammation; Lowers damaging isoprostanes, a byproduct of inflammation.

SELENIUM
Subclinical deficiency negatively alters genes that regulate the inflammatory response; Deficiency promotes vascular inflammation.

Image 27

Improve Cholesterol and Lipids (Image 28)

IMPROVE CHOLESTROL & LIPIDS

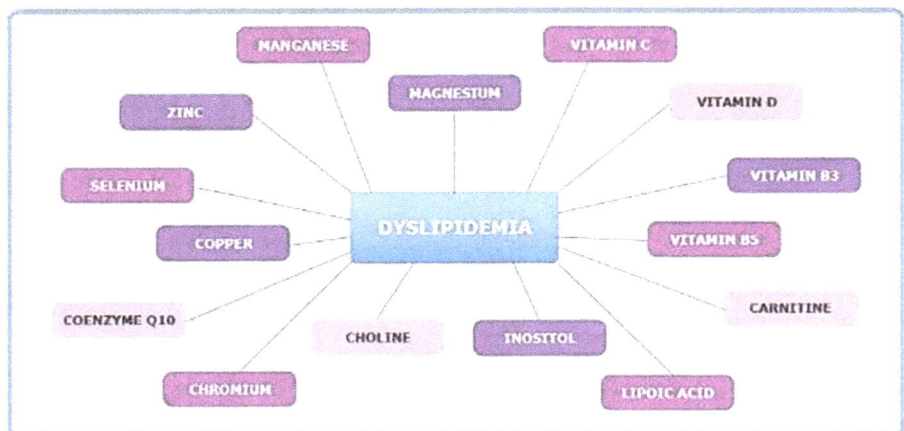

MANGANESE
Cofactor to an antioxidant (superoxide dismutase) that repairs damage to blood vessels caused by oxidized LDL (low density lipoprotein).

MAGNESIUM
Deficiency causes pro-atherogenic (heart-disease causing) changes in lipoprotein metabolism; Protects LDL (low density lipoprotein) from being oxidized.

VITAMIN C
Protects LDL from oxidation, thus making it less "sticky" and prone to atherosclerosis (clogging of arteries); Prevents white blood cells (monocytes) and oxidized LDL from sticking to blood vessel wall; Lowers Lp(a) in some people.

VITAMIN D
Suppresses foam cell formation thus reducing risk of lipid-related arterial blockages; Deficiency linked to dyslipidemia.

VITAMIN B3
Niacin (B3) effectively lowers the highly atherogenic Lp(a) by decreasing its rate of synthesis in the liver.

VITAMIN B5
Favorably alters low density lipoprotein metabolism and reduces triglycerides; Full benefit of lipid lowering effects may not be seen for up to four months.

CARNITINE
In supplementation trials, carnitine lowers triglycerides, oxidized LDL and the atherogenic Lp(a); This effect is likely due to its role in transporting fatty acids into cells so they can be used as fuel.

LIPOIC ACID
Imrpoves lipid profile by reducing small, dense LDL (dangerous type); Protects vascular lining from oxidized cholesterol.

INOSITOL
Decreases small, dense LDL especially in patients with metabolic syndrome; Lowers triglycerides.

CHOLINE
Regulates HDL metabolism; Part of the enzyme lecithin-cholesterol acyltransferase that has a major impact on lipoprotein metabolism.

CHROMIUM
Specifically improves the dyslipidemia that accompanies insulin resistance; May increase HDL; Synergistic effect with niacin (B3) for dyslipidemia.

COENZYME Q10
It is well established that statins, often prescribed for dyslipidemia, deplete CoQ10; Lowers Lp(a) and improves efficacy of some dyslipidemia meds.

COPPER
Several copper-dependent enzymes affect lipoprotein metabolism; Deficiency contributes to fatty buildup in arteries caused by dyslipidemia.

SELENIUM
Prevents post-prandial (after a meal) changes in lipoproteins that make them susceptible to oxidation and thus harmful.

ZINC
Suboptimal zinc raises dangerous lipoproteins that promote vascular inflammation and arterial plaque formation; Cellular zinc controls the gene that makes heart-protective HDL (high density lipoprotein).

Image 28

Prevent and/or Control Diabetes (Image 29)

PREVENT AND/OR CONTROL DIABETES

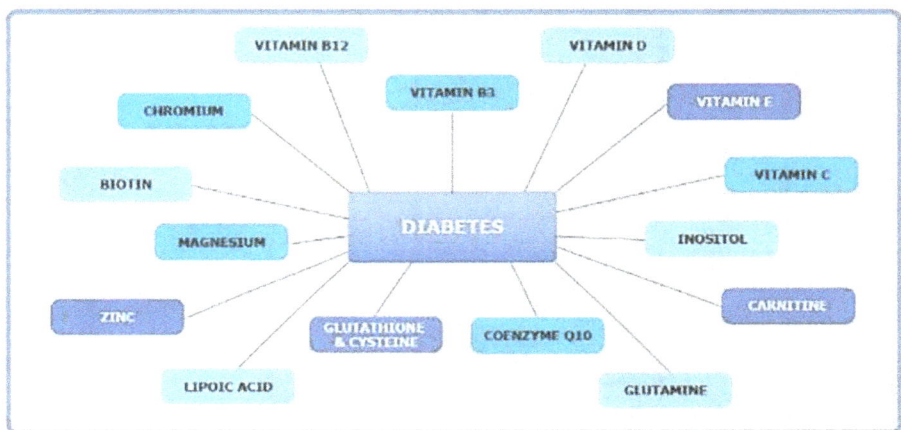

VITAMIN B12
Deficiency common in diabetics because metformin depletes B12.

VITAMIN B3
Preserves B-cell function in type 1 diabetics; Part of GTF (glucose tolerance factor) which facilitates insulin binding.

VITAMIN D
Lowers risk of type 1 and 2 diabetes; Supresses inflammation of pancreatic B-cells; Vitamin D receptor gene linked to diabetes.

VITAMIN E
Confers protection against diabetes by protecting pancreatic B-cells from oxidative stress induced damage; May prevent progression of type I diabetes.

VITAMIN C
Lowers glycosylated hemoglobin (HbAIc) and fasting and post-meal glucose levels and in type 2 diabetics.

INOSITOL
Evidence suggests that inositol may be effective in treating diabetic neuropathy.

CARNITINE
Reduces and even prevents pain from diabetic neuropathy; Improves insulin sensitivity by increasing glucose uptake and storge.

GLUTAMINE
Stimulates a hormone called GLP-I (glucagon-like peptide I) that regulates insulin signaling and sensitivity.

COENZYME Q10
Protects kidney from diabetes related damage; Improves glycemic control in type 2 diabetics.

GLUTATHIONE & CYSTEINE
Glutathione-containing enzymes protect B-cells which are particularly sensitive to oxidative stress; Type 2 diabetics have abnormal antioxidant status; Supplementation with the glutathione precursor cysteine restores antioxidant status.

LIPOIC ACID
Enhances glucose uptake in skeletal muscle tissue; Improves glucose tolerance in type 2 diabetics; Very effective treatment for diabetic neuropathy.

ZINC
Needed in the synthesis, storage and secretion of insulin; Protects pancreatic B-cells from damage; Affects the expression of genes linked to diabetes.

MAGNESIUM
Deficiency reduces insulin sensitivity; Low magnesium exacerbates foot ulcers in diabetics.

BIOTIN

Stimulates glucose-induced insulin secretion in pancreatic B-cells; High dose biotin can improve glycemic control in diabetics.

CHROMIUM
Helps insulin attach to cell's receptors increasing glucose uptake into cell; Supplementation trials show dose-dependent benefits for type II diabetics

Image 29

Manage Hypertension (Image 30)

MANAGE HYPERTENSION

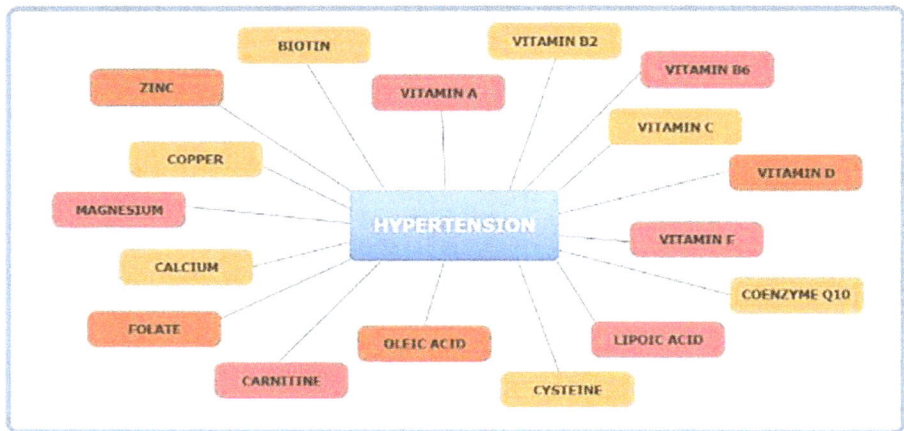

Biotin
Pharmacological doses reduce systolic blood pressure by activating an enzyme (cGMP) that causes smooth muscle to relax.

Vitamin A
Suppresses the growth of vascular smooth muscle, thus keeping blood vessels (lumen) clear and wide.

Vitamin B2
People with a certain gene (called MTHFR type TT) tend to respond well to B2 therapy for lowering blood pressure.

Vitamin B6
Lowers homocysteine, a toxin that makes arteries stiff and raises blood pressure; Low B6 is strongly linked to hypertension.

Vitamin C
Improves the ability of blood vessels to react appropriately to relaxation signals; Increases nitric oxide, a powerful vasodilator.

Vitamin D
Low vitamin D is strongly linked to hypertension, possibly due to its role in calcium transport; Augments blood pressure lowering effect of calcium; Keeps blood vessels smooth and healthy.

Vitamin E
Increases nitric oxide synthase, an enzyme that causes blood vessels to dilate; Protects blood vessels from damage.

Coenzyme Q10
Improves bioenergetics of blood vessel wall; Deficiency highly correlated to hypertension; Benefits of CoQ10 often not seen for several weeks.

Lipoic Acid
Improves vascular tone; Causes vasodilation; Works like calcium channel blocker meds; Recycles vitamins C, E and cysteine.

Cysteine Anti-hypertensive effects stem from its role as a potent antioxidant; Effective vasodilator.

Oleic Acid The benefits of olive oil for blood pressure are largely due to its high oleic acid content, which protects endothelial cells (inner lining of blood vessels) from inflammation.

Carnitine Lowers blood pressure in the same way as ACE inhibitors, a common hypertension drug which reduces angiotensin, a substance that causes arteries to constrict; Its role in fat metabolism explains this effect.

Folate Lowers blood pressure by improving endothelial function, or the ability of blood vessels to properly dilate.

Calcium Optimal calcium status reduces vasoconstriction; Particularly effective for salt-sensitive hypertension as it increases sodium excretion.

Magnesium Promotes dilation of blood vessels; Low intracellular levels are a well established cause of hypertension.

Copper Regulates enzymes that keep blood vessels dilating properly; Depletion causes hypertension; Supplementation trials positive.

Zinc Regulates angiotensin and endothelin, two enzymes that directly affect blood pressure; Deficiency causes blood vessels to constrict.

Image 30

Improve Metabolic Status (Image 31)

IMPROVE METABOLIC STATUS

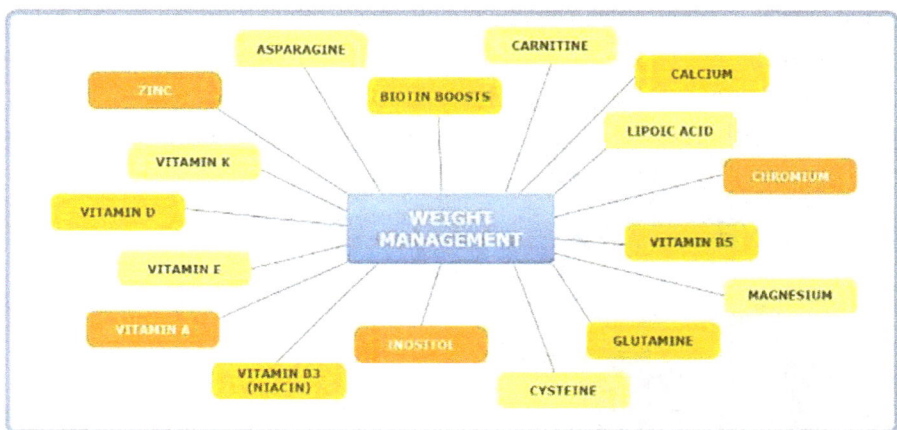

ASPARAGINE
This amino acid increases insulin sensitivity which helps the body store energy in muscle instead of storing it as body fat.

BIOTIN BOOSTS
metabolism by improving glycemic control (stabilizes blood sugar) and lowering insulin, a hormone that promotes fat formation.

CARNITINE
Carries fatty acids into the cell so they can be burned for fuel; Helps reduce visceral adiposity (belly fat)

CALCIUM
Inhibits the formation of fat cells; Also helps oxidize (burn) fat cells.

LIPOIC ACID
Improves glucose uptake into cells, which helps a person burn carbohydrates more efficiently.

CHROMIUM
Makes the body more sensitive to insulin, helping to reduce body fat and increase lean muscle.

VITAMIN B5
Taking B5 lowers body weight by activating lipoprotein lipase, an enzyme that burns fat cells. One study liked B5 supplementation to less hunger when dieting.

MAGNESIUM
Low magnesium in cells impairs a person's ability to use glucose for fuel, instead storing it as fat; Correcting a magnesium deficiency stimulates metabolism by increasing insulin sensitivity. Magnesium may also inhibit fat absorption.

GLUTAMINE
Reduces fat mass by improving glucose uptake into muscle.

CYSTEINE
Supplementation with this antioxidant reduced body fat in obese patients.

INOSITOL
Supplementation may increase adiponectin levels.

VITAMIN B3 (NIACIN)
Treatment with B3 increases adiponectin, a weight-loss hormone secreted by fat cells; Niacin-bound chromium supplements helped reduced body weight in clinical trials.

VITAMIN A
Enhances expression of genes that reduce a person's tendency to store food as fat; reduces the size of fat cells.

VITAMIN E
Inhibits pre-fat cells from changing into mature fat cells, thus reducing body fat.

VITAMIN D
Deficiency strongly linked to poor metabolism of carbohydrates; Genes that are regulated by vitamin D may alter the way fat cells form in some people.

VITAMIN K
Poor vitamin K status linked to excess fat tissue; vitamin K helps metabolize sugars.

ZINC
Deficiency of zinc reduces leptin, a beneficial hormone that regulates appetites, which is reversed by zinc repletion

Image 31

Exercise

Another critical aspect to healthy living, wellness, and improved health outcomes includes Exercise. The Wellness VIP Patient portal provides improved insight to individuals with an earnest desire to make positive changes. Upon selecting 'Exercise' from the top menu, patients are presented with additional resources which may help them in their quest for improved health outcomes (Image 32).

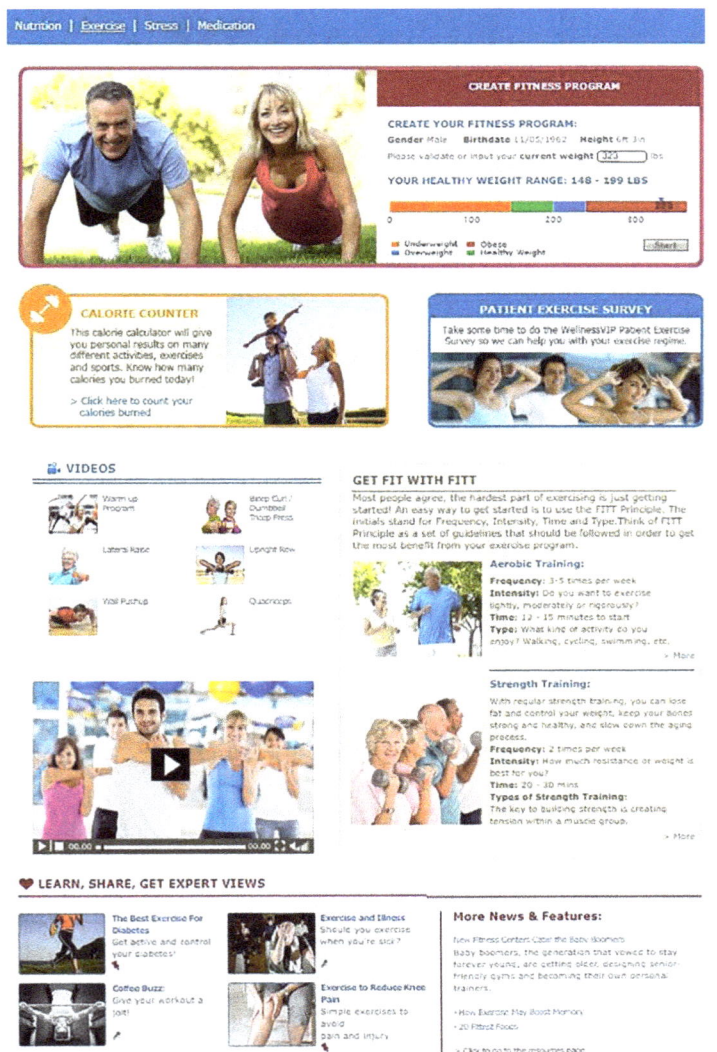

Image 32

A Calorie Counter and Exercise Activity calculator is provided to help patients identify the number of calories burned for each type of exercise performed. These calories are calculated based on the patient's individual biometric data. After looking up the number of calories that are burned for a wide range of physical activities, the patient can log that activity in their daily activity diary with the simple touch of a button. The diary then tracks the patient's performance over time (Image 33).

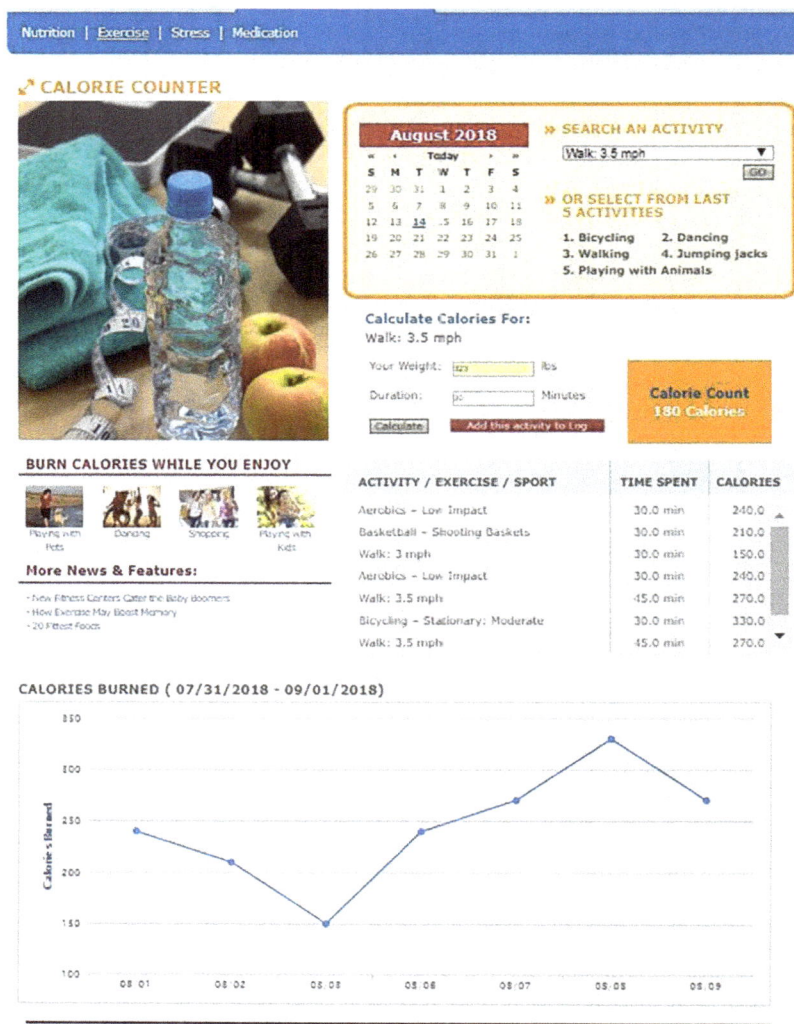

Image 33

A Patient Exercise Survey is provided to assist the health care profession in providing relevant exercise and activity guidance (Image 34).

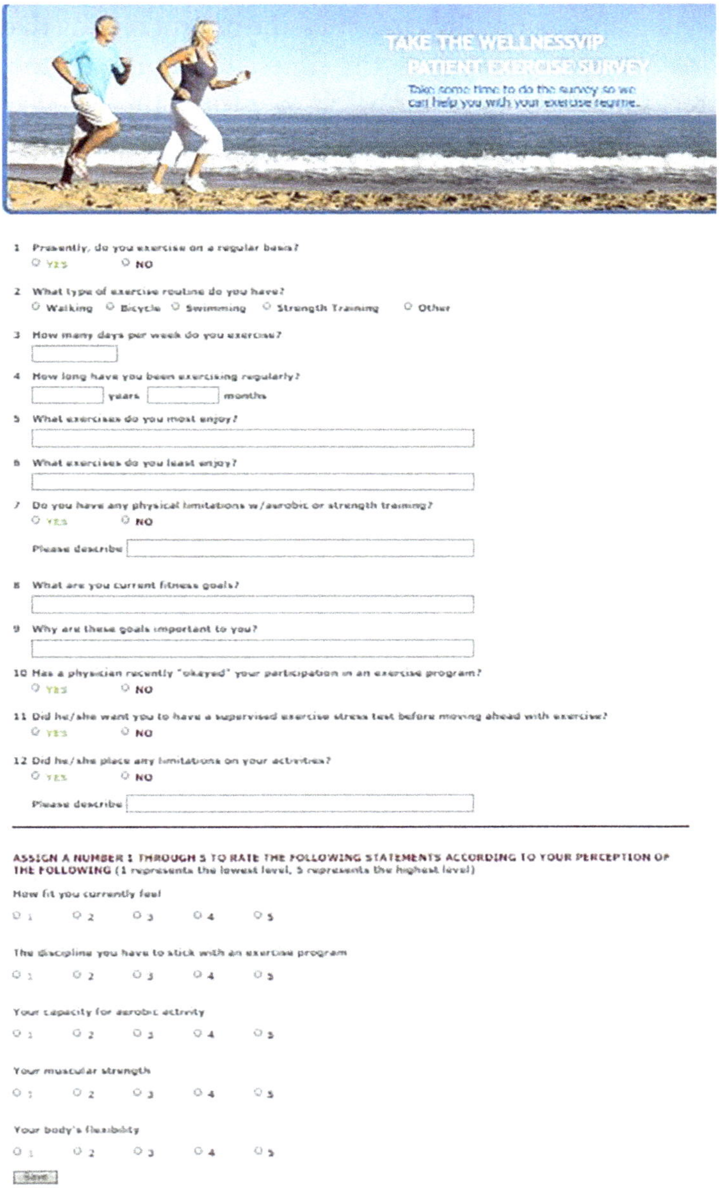

1 Presently, do you exercise on a regular basis?
   ○ YES   ○ NO

2 What type of exercise routine do you have?
   ○ Walking   ○ Bicycle   ○ Swimming   ○ Strength Training   ○ Other

3 How many days per week do you exercise?

4 How long have you been exercising regularly?
   _____ years   _____ months

5 What exercises do you most enjoy?

6 What exercises do you least enjoy?

7 Do you have any physical limitations w/aerobic or strength training?
   ○ YES   ○ NO

   Please describe

8 What are you current fitness goals?

9 Why are these goals important to you?

10 Has a physician recently "okayed" your participation in an exercise program?
   ○ YES   ○ NO

11 Did he/she want you to have a supervised exercise stress test before moving ahead with exercise?
   ○ YES   ○ NO

12 Did he/she place any limitations on your activities?
   ○ YES   ○ NO

   Please describe

ASSIGN A NUMBER 1 THROUGH 5 TO RATE THE FOLLOWING STATEMENTS ACCORDING TO YOUR PERCEPTION OF THE FOLLOWING (1 represents the lowest level, 5 represents the highest level)

How fit you currently feel
○ 1   ○ 2   ○ 3   ○ 4   ○ 5

The discipline you have to stick with an exercise program
○ 1   ○ 2   ○ 3   ○ 4   ○ 5

Your capacity for aerobic activity
○ 1   ○ 2   ○ 3   ○ 4   ○ 5

Your muscular strength
○ 1   ○ 2   ○ 3   ○ 4   ○ 5

Your body's flexibility
○ 1   ○ 2   ○ 3   ○ 4   ○ 5

[Save]

Image 34

Additional guidance is provided using the FITT methodology (e.g. Frequency, Intensity, Time, and Type). This method has been proven to be effective at guiding compliant patients to improved health outcomes. FITT is an easy way to think about exercise and activity. The FITT guidance is provided for both Aerobic activity (Image 35) and for Strength Training (Image 36).

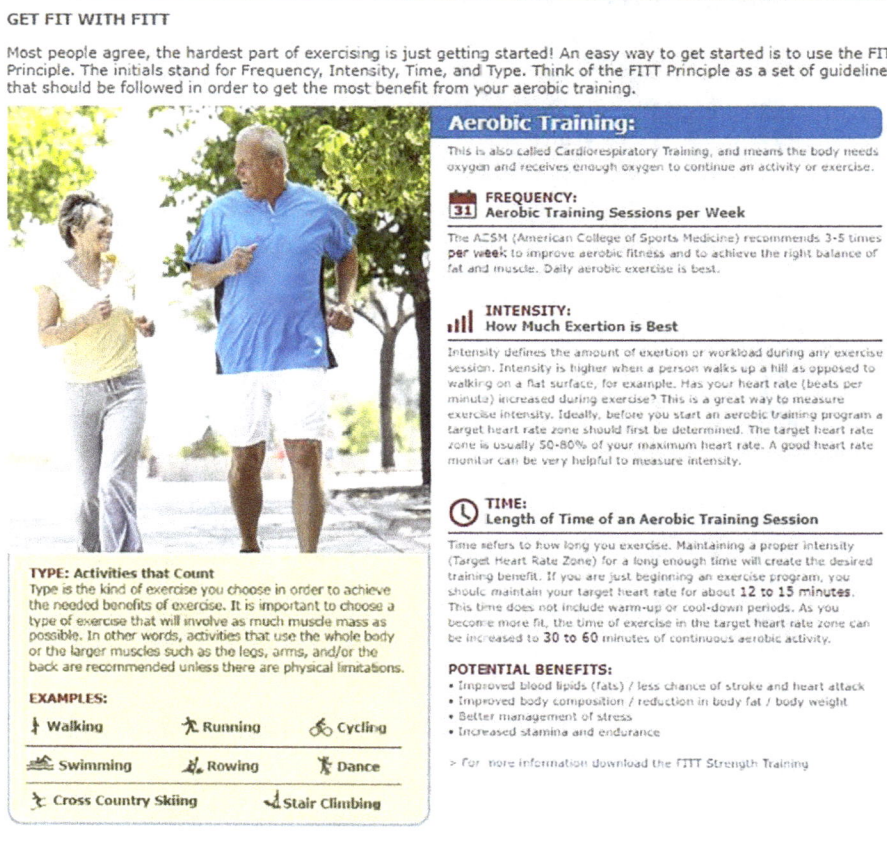

Image 35

Nutrition | Exercise | Stress | Medication

GET FIT WITH FITT

Most people agree, the hardest part of exercising is just getting started! An easy way to get started is to use the FITT Principle. The initials stand for Frequency, Intensity, Time, and Type. Think of the FITT Principle as a set of guidelines that should be followed in order to get the most benefit from your aerobic training.

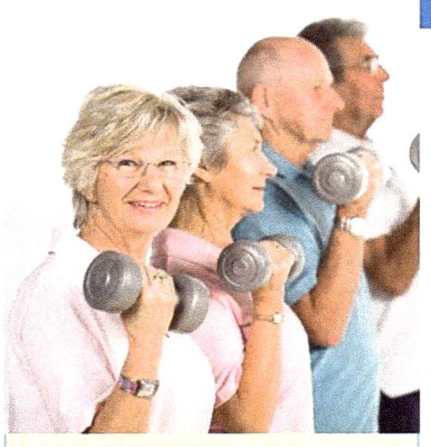

Strength Training:

Most people are unaware that strenth training is an important part of a complete fitness program. Not only can you increase your strength by more than 50 percent in just 2 months with regular strength training, you can lose fat and control your weight, keep your bones strong and healthy, and slow down the aging process! And...the more muscle you have, the more calories you burn at rest and during exercise!! To get the best benefit from strength training, keep in mind the FITT Principle (Frequency, Intensity, Time, Type)

FREQUENCY:
31 Number of Strength Training Sessions per Week

• Aim to train each muscle group at least 2 times per week, and up to three if you have the time or are used to strength training. One day per week may help you maintain your current level of strength, but it will not be enough to build muscle.

• It is important to rest 1 to 2 days in between working out the same muscle(s). Rest days are needed to give the muscles time to recover and become stronger.

INTENSITY:
How Much Weight/Resistance is Best

This can be a tricky one – and if you're new to exercise, it will take some trial and error. The intensity of the resistance should challenge you. It should be high enough that as you approach your last repetition, you feel your muscles getting tired. For strength training, workload is the main measure of intensity during exercise and can have three components:

1. The amount of weight lifted during exercise.
2. The number of repetitions completed for a particular exercise.
3. The length of time to complete all exercises in a set or total training aalsession.

TIME:
Length of time to strength train

The total time of a strength training session will vary depending on how fit you are. The minimal commitment for strength training is 20 to 30 minutes per workout 2 times a week. When beginning strength training, it is recommended that there be no more than 2 to 3 minutes between sets of exercises. As you become more fit, decrease your time to 1 minute between each set.

POTENTIAL BENEFITS:
• Fat loss, Weight Control and Weight Maintenance
• Increased Metabolism
• Increased Stamina and Endurance
• Increased Muscle Mass and Overall Strength

> For more information download the FITT Strength Training

TYPES OF STRENGTH TRAINING:

The most important thing to remember is the Tension Principle:

Deltoids   Pectorals

Obliques

Biceps

Upper Abdominals

Lower Abdominals   Quadriceps

The key to building strength is creating tension within a muscle group. Tension is created by resistance. Resistance can come from weights (dumbbells or free weights), specially designed machines (Nautilus®, Paramount®, Cybex®, etc.), resistance bands, or the weight of your own body.

Exercise every major muscle group (arms, chest, back, core, and legs) when strength training. Make sure you work opposing muscles, not just the ones you see when you look in the mirror.

Image 36

Fitness videos are also included to help guide patients through various types of exercises (Image 37). This information is particularly helpful for individuals and patients who are novices and just beginning to exercise regularly.

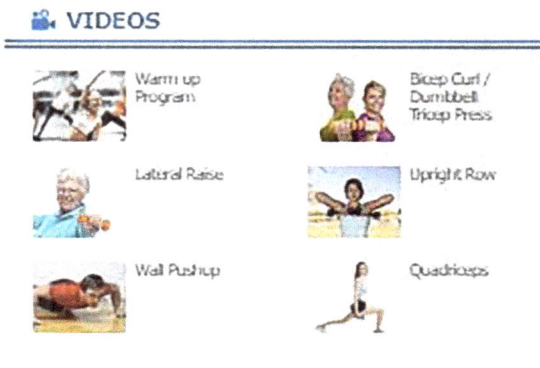

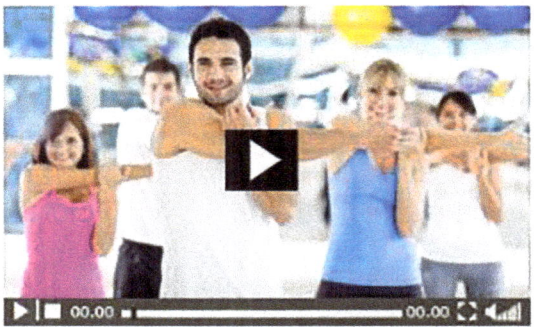

Image 37

Additional resources and links to exercises, exercise websites and articles which promote healthy habits and wellness are provided and updated periodically (Image 38).

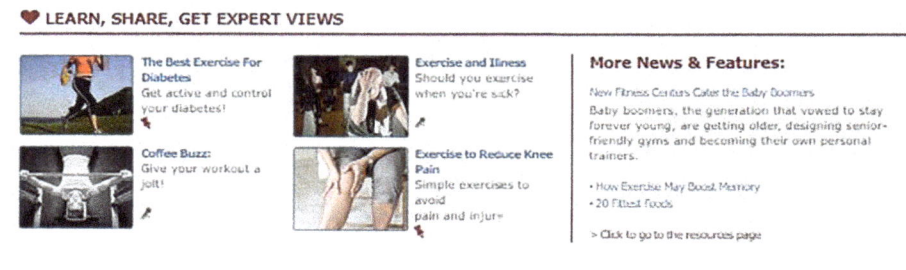

Image 38

CONCLUSION

The Wellness VIP Patient Portal is a robust integrated tool which links patients with their primary care providers. The Patient Portal provides patients with direct access to their personalized treatment plans, the results from their most recent and historical testing, and the tools to help them more effectively implement and be successful at maintaining and complying with the health directives agreed upon with their health providers.

Perhaps more importantly, this comprehensive program is available to both patients and providers at no cost. That's right – we created the program to be available to the patients of our providers who actively use our program. Since there is **<u>no cost</u>** to the provider OR the patient for joining the VIP program, only a commitment to implement its principles into the practice – there should be no reason that would prevent a practitioner from getting involved with the Wellness VIP Program.

If you are a physician, I urge you to contact CardioRisk Laboratories to learn how easy it is to be a Wellness VIP provider. If you are a patient, I urge you to put your primary care provider in touch with us or give them a copy of this book. The opportunity cost of NOT taking action might be your good health and wellness.

FUNCTION

There are over 60,000 miles of vasculature in the human body. Over 90% of these vessels are microvascular and barely visible with the human eye. Vascular function, and more specifically, endothelial function is the most important part of vascular health.

The most obvious answer for why one should consider adding a test to measure vascular function is because that is obviously where the action of cardiovascular disease takes place. Vascular function testing provides a weather gauge for cardiovascular risk. It provides an integrated index which summarizes the cumulative effects of cardiovascular risk factors and those cardio-protective factors active in patients.

In short, vascular function testing provides important insight into the effects of patient's health habits such as smoking, and their risk conditions such as diabetes, hypertension, genetics, and aging. It can also provide valuable insight into patient's healthy habits such as activity (or the lack thereof), diet, cholesterol, oxidative stress, and the effects of pharmacological interventions.

Vascular function takes place in the endothelium, a single cell thick membrane that is the largest organ in the body. It lines every vessel and every organ in the body. The vascular endothelium serves several crucial functions relating to cardiovascular disease. First, it functions very much like a Teflon coating in that it acts as a semi-selective barrier between the vessel lumen and the surrounding tissue. It literally controls the passage of materials and the transit of white blood cells into and out of the bloodstream. Excessive or even prolonged increases in the permeability of this layer can lead to chronic inflammation and could lead to tissue edema or swelling.

The vascular endothelium regulates the traffic of fluids and molecules between blood and tissues. This is important since the atherosclerotic process can't take place without vascular wall penetration and the subsequent inflammatory process. The vascular endothelium plays a vital role in vascular tone and in the regulation of blood flow which contributes to vascular homeostasis and repair. This can include the formation of new blood vessels as in angiogenesis.

When healthy, it is involved in the repair of damaged or diseased organs via an injection of blood vessel cells. The endothelium will normally provide a non-stick (or non-thrombogenic) surface because, when healthy, it contains heparan sulfate which acts as a cofactor for activating antithrombin. This protease inactivates several of the factors directly involved in the cascade leading to coagulation. So, in its role as an anti-coagulant service it prevents certain pathogens from aggregation and even penetration into the intima and media layers of the vessel.

Vascular dysfunction provides one of the earliest indications that a patient is progressing towards vascular disease. Over time, pathogens such as cholesterol penetrate and perforate this thin wall. Once compromised, a series of unhealthy conditions manifest creating a range of vascular sequelae including inflammation and culminating in full atherosclerotic plaque buildup, subsequent thrombus, and often clinical events.

Because the endothelium is a crucial membrane which affects virtually every organ and most of the body's systems, its importance to good health cannot be overstated. Endothelial dysfunction has been associated with Sleep Apnea, Raynaud's Disease, Stroke, Dementia, Macular Degeneration Alzheimer's Disease, Periodontal Disease, Erectile Dysfunction, Peripheral Arterial Disease, Pulmonary Hypertension, Angina, Heart Failure, Heart Attack, Renal Failure, Pre-Eclampsia, Diabetes, Portal Hypertension and Hypertension. Clinicians often find evidence of vascular or endothelial dysfunction in their practice.

A compromised endothelium, as manifest by endothelial dysfunction or the loss of healthy endothelial function, is a diagnostic hallmark of vascular diseases. Deteriorated or impaired endothelial function is a leading cause behind hypertension and thrombosis. This is almost always seen in coronary arterial disease, diabetes mellitus, and even hypercholesterolemia. It has been shown to be predictive of future cardiovascular events, rheumatoid arthritis, and systemic lupus erythematosus.

The image below (Image 39) (Naghavi, 2017) captures an overview of the progression of scientific knowledge surrounding vascular function and leading to the scientific rationale for active monitoring of vascular function in a clinical setting.

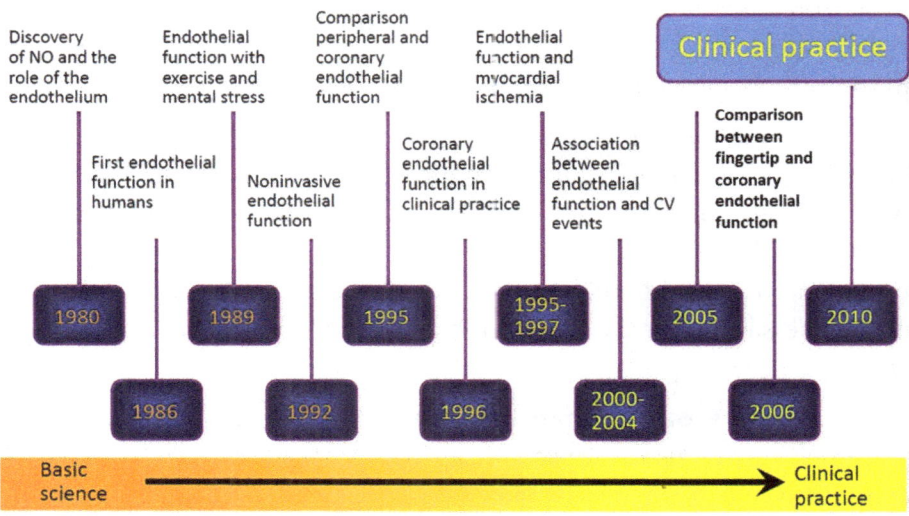

Image 39

Example of Vascular Function

While the exact mechanisms of vascular function are only mildly understood, there is one example that is familiar to virtually anyone who has undergone an aggressive exercise routine and experience the phenomenon known as the *second wind*. While there are undoubtedly many factors which contribute to the effect of this phenomenon, at least one of those is related to vascular function.

When a person begins a long run, they inevitably experience shortness of breath as their body's physiology tries to 'catch up' to the level of activity that was suddenly imposed upon it. Essentially the heart screams to the brain "I need air". The brain verifies this fact and sends a signal to the vessel(s) affected by the increased exertion (in this case the heart) and tells the vessels to release nitric oxide (NO). Nitric oxide is a colorless gas and free radical which is stored in vessels throughout the body. Its release triggers vasodilation which, of course, increases the amount of blood flow to the area of interest . . . and a concurrent increase in oxygen to the affected area(s).

Although this example is a gross over simplification of the process – that vasodilation resulting from the release of NO contributes at least partially to the phenomenon known as "the second wind" is indisputable.

As we age, and particularly as lifestyle and other factors which contribute to the damage of the endothelium layer continue – this thin wall gets compromised. Pathogens such as cholesterol and other radicals poke holes in its fragile surface and this has the net affect of pouring water on a circuit board. The net effect of the damaged endothelium is that messages to release NO don't get where they are supposed to go, when they are supposed to go.

The cascade of other protective factors which are affected by the endothelium are also compromised. This leads to a myriad of chronic conditions which eventually will almost always affect the vasculature in some clinically manifestation.

If you ever watch late night television, you will likely be bombarded with an assortment of advertisements for men for vasodilators like Viagra and Cialis which treat erectile dysfunction. These medications help to treat an extremely common condition in men over 50. The problem is largely one of vascular function. The very name is suggestive of this fact: *Erectile Dysfunction* or *ED*. Erectile Dysfunction occurs when the signals that release nitric oxide to cause vasodilation don't get to the right place at the right time. In the case of ED, we rarely know if the condition is resulting from a pharmacologically induced dysfunction from some medication the patient may be taking; or whether it is a psychological condition which led to emasculation or some other psychologically induced sequelae; the final reason could be a physiological condition. Endothelial Function testing can tell us definitively if the patient's physiology is functioning correctly.

The reasons to test the endothelium and vascular function should be obvious by now. Clinically, endothelium and vascular testing provide one of the earliest indicators of atherosclerosis and other vascular conditions. Since testing can be completed at your office in a relatively inexpensive, safe and non-invasive manner – requiring no needle sticks or disrobing. . . it is one of the 3 steps that can help you to minimize cardio and cerebrovascular events in your practice. Let's look at some of the ways this can be accomplished.

Testing Modalities for Endothelial Function

One of the two changes I'm recommending you make is to add CardioRisk's EndoTherm™ testing into your routine practice. EndoTherm™ is a simple non-invasive technology which measures the strength and speed of a post-occlusive reactive hyperemia. Similar technologies are available which use amplitude signal (such as the EndoPAT). These can create confounding data by creating impedance or amplitude signals when patients move their fingers.

The EndoTherm™ uses digital temperature measurements at the microvasculature of the fingertips. These measurements capture the strength and speed of the temperature rebound following an occlusion of the brachial artery. The test is differentiated from Ankle Brachial Index and other Flow Mediated Dilation or Plethsymography tests in that each patient provides the ideal control for their test population (n) of 1.

The test is customarily performed on each patient's right arm, and their left arm is used as a control. This control is an important differentiator because it allows us to examine each individual and compare themselves against their perfect comparative standard (e.g. the patient's left arm compared to their right arm), rather than a population or epidemiologic database.

Since the patient's left arm is left untouched during the period where the right arm is occluded, it provides a unique and patient specific range of normal. The cuffing of the right arm provides enough stress to stimulate the release of nitric oxide (NO) causing a post occlusive vasodilation or reactive hyperemia.

The strength and speed of this response is measured and compared to the control arm. The subsequent calculation provides a predictable and consistent response index which can be used to compare patient's improvement over time. In other words – the test can be an important data point to guide therapy and patient health outcome goals.

The test had been correlated with higher coronary plaque burden (Eldredge, 2016), a higher burden of cardiovascular risk factors measured by Framingham Risk Score, high coronary artery calcium score, and the presence of cardiometabolic disorders. It has been shown to improve the identification of high risk diabetic patients and has been associated with increased insulin resistance.

All tests have their weaknesses, and the EndoTherm™ is no different. Because blood pressure cuffs are inflated bilaterally, patient's who have had a mastectomy or other surgical procedure which could impair the vessels surrounding the brachial tree should not have this test.

Also, the test can be uncomfortable for fragile patients. The occlusion period is five minutes, and this can make some patients anxious and cause a tingling sensation or dull ache which a small number of patients cannot tolerate. CardioRisk technicians will terminate the test if a patient complains of any sharp pain or dizziness. Although I'm not aware of this ever happening in thousands of endothelial function tests we've preformed, precautionary measures should be in place just in case.

Finally, because this is a physiological test, it is highly recommended that the patients fast from food and sugary or caffeinated drinks for 8 hours (but at least 4 hours) prior to the testing time. It is well known that fingertip temperatures are affected by autonomic nervous system activity. Usually, the higher the sympathetic activity, the lower the fingertip temperature. Although the software controls for these variations – care should be taken to minimize activities that affect the autonomic nervous system. Patients should stay away from medications which would cause vasodilation for at least a complete half-life or 24 hours. All other medications should be taken as prescribed because the test is optimally conducted while patients are in their most steady state.

WHAT CAN I DO ABOUT VASCULAR DYSFUNCTION?

The good news is that we have known how to treat and even repair the endothelium, so we don't have to accept a compromised vascular wall even in our elderly patients. One of the important effects of the statin class of drugs has long been its proven ability to repair the endothelial wall surface, this in addition to its better-known cholesterol lowering benefits (Dimmeler, 2001), (Besler, 2014), (DelPapa, 2008), (Naruszewicz, 2008).

Exercise and a healthy lifestyle are important mediators of vascular function.

TAKE AWAYS:

Adding this one test will help you to identify patients in the very earliest stages of disease, allowing you time to treat them medically. EndoTherm™ vascular function testing takes less than 30 minutes, requires no needle sticks or disrobing, and is often covered by 3rd party payers. Whether or not the procedure is covered for your patient should not be a barrier to offering them the test.

Adult patients will benefit by knowing the strength of their vascular function. The test is an important motivator that will help change patient behavior relating to lifestyle as it is a direct indicator of exercise physiology. Perhaps most importantly, the test is reproducible and effective at monitoring physiological changes over time.

STRUCTURE

There a number of technologies we could put under this header. The concept behind structural wall testing is simple, it is a superior technology to either of the other two methods (e.g. blood and function). If you are only going to make one change to your practice, let it be the implementation of structural wall testing to your screening and monitoring practice.

At the time that we stick a needle into your vein and draw some blood out, not one drop of it has hurt you. Let's be clear, as it relates to cardiovascular disease, the pathogens found in the blood must penetrate the one-cell thick layer of the endothelium before they can begin causing problems which will subsequently lead to inflammation and atherosclerosis. So, at the time that we draw blood out of your vein, the best we can do is measure the concentration of a pathogen per deciliter of blood or some other measurement equivalent. This was explained more completely in the chapter on blood. When we look at cholesterol and other traditional blood tests, we are measuring the probability that a certain concentration of pathogens will eventually cause problems in the structural wall of the vessel.

The advantage of testing a patient's structural walls is that we bypass all the probabilities of damage to those vessels. With structural testing we are directly measuring the amount of disease in the arterial wall. It's like a pregnancy test for heart disease.

This method doesn't care how you got it. It doesn't care whether it is a concentration of some pathogen in the blood, a lifestyle shortcoming, a genetic predisposition, an environmental factor, or any other cause . . . it just tells you whether you have atherosclerosis in the wall of the artery. Some of these tests can tell you if there is any active inflammation that would precede an atherosclerotic lesion.

There are over 250 known risk factors for cardiovascular disease. The real beauty of structural wall screening is that it doesn't matter which, or how many of these variables apply to you or your patient . . . the structural wall tests will tell you definitively if any of those risk factors has had a systemic effect. The more people you can catch with disease early on in its pathophysiological pathway, the more people you can prevent from experiencing a clinical event.

Some of the structural tests available to you include: MRI, Coronary Calcium Score (CAC), IVUS, Angiography, CIMT, and Carotid Duplex exams. Outlined below is a recommendation for one test that can easily be added to your routine practice.

CAROTID AND/OR FEMORAL IMT

If you are only going to implement one concept from this book, let it be the addition of routine Intima Media Thickness (IMT) testing into your practice. The data is so compelling that my jaw often drops when confronted by the occasional 'nay-sayer'. As there are for virtually any medical procedure, there are people on both sides of the fence. IMT, and specifically CIMT is no different. Having said that, I have attempted to directly address both sides of the argument.

Let's begin with what I believe is the most compelling piece of data currently available regarding this technology. In the year 2000, a group of researchers published what could be considered the most important data ever produced on the efficacy of this technology. The study was a randomized prospective study from a population in Italy (Belcaro, 2001). The same 10,000 patients were followed for 10 years. That is a large 100,000-person-year study. They don't come much larger.

At the onset of the study, prospective participants were screened and eliminated if they had any cardiovascular, renal, metabolic problems, or genetic diseases. The researchers eliminated the higher risk patients to get a cohort of low-risk participants. This was important because they planned to simply watch these patients over time without treatment. At the time of the study the efficacy of IMT was uncertain, so the prospect of monitoring 10,000 low-risk patients to observe and measure the progression or lack of progression of arterial disease in their arteries seemed prudent. Each of the participants signed waivers and agreed to have no treatment, regardless of what was found in their arteries.

What happened was simply stunning. 21% of that population went on to experience clinical events within the 10-year time window of the study. The net results were this: 1) IMT (both carotid and femoral) correctly identified 98.6 of those who went on to have events as having increased risk. 2) Only 1 in 800 of those found to have 'normal' arteries went on to have an event.

Think about the ramification of that in your practice. What if you could successfully identify and take prescriptive measures for 98.6% of YOUR patients who could go on to have a Heart Attack or Stroke? A home pregnancy test catches about 97% for heaven's sake (Bastian, 1998).

I challenge you to find ANY test in your toolbox that has been shown to catch a higher percentage of those who go on to have events. I haven't' found one!

So what about false positives you ask? To that I would ask you, "what constitutes a false positive in your mind?" if you are asking whether or not every patient that was identified as having an increased risk for an event goes on to have an event, I would tell you that 'no, of course not'. What test do you have in your toolbox now that does that? Not blood. Not function. Certainly not the Framingham or alternative risk screening tools. The answer is that none of them do.

We must remember that only 1 out of 800 of the group that had normal vessels went on to have an event in the 10-year window. We also must consider that the study only looked at a 10-year window. This doesn't mean that those who were flagged as having abnormal arteries were without risk, just that they didn't have an event in that time frame. Indeed, we now understand that patients with plaque have the same risk of a future event as those who have already had one (Naqvi, 2014). In this study, 51 out of 61 in the highest risk class had an event in the 10-year window. 239 out of 611 patients in the second highest risk class went on to have events in that 10-year window.

Those in the higher risk groups that did not go on to experience a clinical event in the 10-year horizon were not disease free. We certainly could not get comfortable or ethically justify not offering them aggressive treatment given the amount of disease found in their arteries and the subsequent risk of experiencing a clinical event.

The idea is to find more people with disease in time to treat them medically so that you don't need to treat them surgically down the road.

That is the only way we can significantly reduce the morbidity and mortality of this disease.

Another data point is the landmark Atherosclerosis Risk in Communities Study (ARIC) (Chambless, 1997). This study looked at a large swath of data which is still referred to today to guide policy risk stratification. There are hundreds of papers published regarding the ARIC data set. One of the original papers which looked at the correlation between IMT and other traditional risk factors found something that is also exciting but often overlooked.

When looking at the Hazard Risk Ratios from various markers, they found the following: an increased LDL level $\geq$ 160 mg/dL created a hazard risk ratio of just 2.01 in women and 1.63 for men. Extremely high LDL concentrations essentially doubled the lifetime risk for women and increased it by 63% in men. An extremely low HDL level $\leq$ 35 resulted in a hazard risk ratio of 4.65 in women and 2.24 in men. Now we are getting somewhere. Women with extremely low HDL levels had a four-fold increase in risk compared to women with 'normal' levels and even in men, the risk more than doubled.

Now the drum roll please. Patients with an IMT measurement $\geq$ 1.0mm (an extremely common occurrence in my experience) resulted in a hazard risk ratio of 18.93 in women and 4.22 in men. Wow! In this cohort, women's lifetime risk increased 19-fold if they have an IMT $\geq$ 1.0mm vs those who had 'normal' arteries. That is a nine-fold increase in risk prediction when compared to LDL and over a five-fold increase in risk when compared to HDL.

The risk ratios for stroke were similar (Chambless, 2000). Females with IMT measurements $\geq$ 1.0mm had a risk ratio of 8.54 when compared to females with normal IMT measurements. Men with IMT measurements $\geq$ 1.0mm had a risk ratio of 3.64 when compared to men with normal IMT measurements.

This data is compelling and should underscore the utility of using IMT to routinely screen adult patients for cardiovascular disease. There are over 10,000 studies which speak to the utility of this single screening tool.

IMT has been used by the FDA as a surrogate end-point for nearly 40 years. Clear back in the year 2000, the American Heart Association's (AHA) expert panel concluded that: "Carotid artery B-mode ultrasound imaging is a safe, noninvasive, and relatively inexpensive means of assessing subclinical atherosclerosis. The technique is a valid and reliable means of measuring IMT, an operational measure of atherosclerosis. The severity of carotid IMT is an independent predictor of transient cerebral ischemia, stroke, and coronary events such as MI." (Greenland, 2000)

This recommendation was not reached haphazardly – it was reached by pouring over hundreds of studies, many of them landmark epidemiological studies which, like many of the studies referred to above, clearly demonstrate the utility of the technology.

As the FDA used IMT to monitor the effect of treatment over time relating to a particular medication, so can the primary care provider utilize it to monitor the effect(s) of treatment on their patients. While the use in a clinical setting is significantly different than a prospective well-controlled trial, especially as it relates to the addition of potential confounders, it does provide unique insight into the patient's arterial vessels which cannot be evaluated any other way. Using CIMT to monitor efficacy of treatment of disease over time, or simply the disease's progression in the untreated patient over time can provide confidence in the prescribed treatment plan, or conversely, inform the provider of the need for more aggressive therapy.

Let's take a look at why this information can be useful.

What is IMT?

A normal artery has 3 distinct layers: the intima, which is the innermost layer and is composed of a single layer of endothelial cells on the luminal surface; the media, a tube of vascular smooth muscle cells and their extracellular matrix; and the adventitia, the outer protective layer made up of loose connective tissue which holds the blood vessels and nerves that supply the artery itself. The adventitia maintains the basement membrane and modifying lipoproteins as they cross into the arterial wall. (Image 40) (Ross R. , 1993)

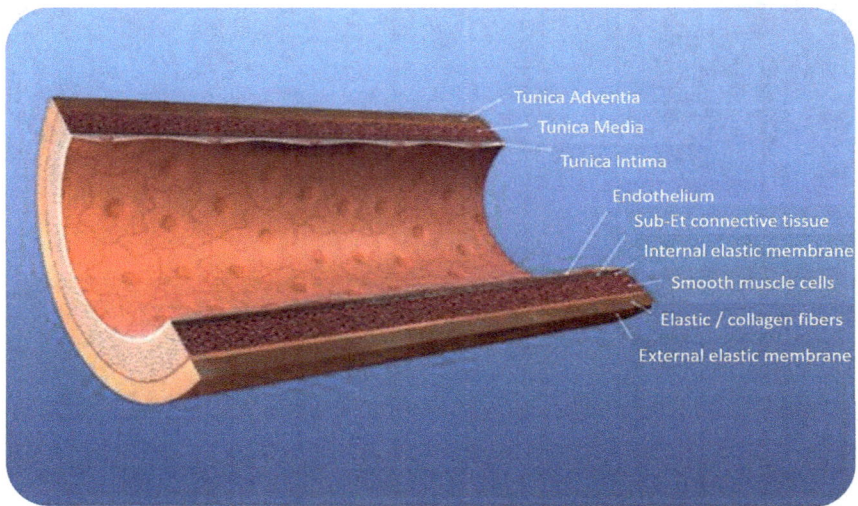

Image 40

Vascular smooth muscle cells of the media contract and relax to change the diameter of the vessel lumen in response to a variety of local stimuli which circulates in the blood. These stimuli regulate vascular tone, blood flow, and blood pressure. Regulation is caused by the production of several vasoactive substances, including prostaglandins, endothelin, and nitric oxide (NO).

The IMT exam consists of measuring the intima and media layers of the artery (Image 41), which can be visualized in B-Mode ultrasound as the area between the black or darkest area of the lumen and the bright white signal of the adventitia (shown in yellow on Image 42 below).

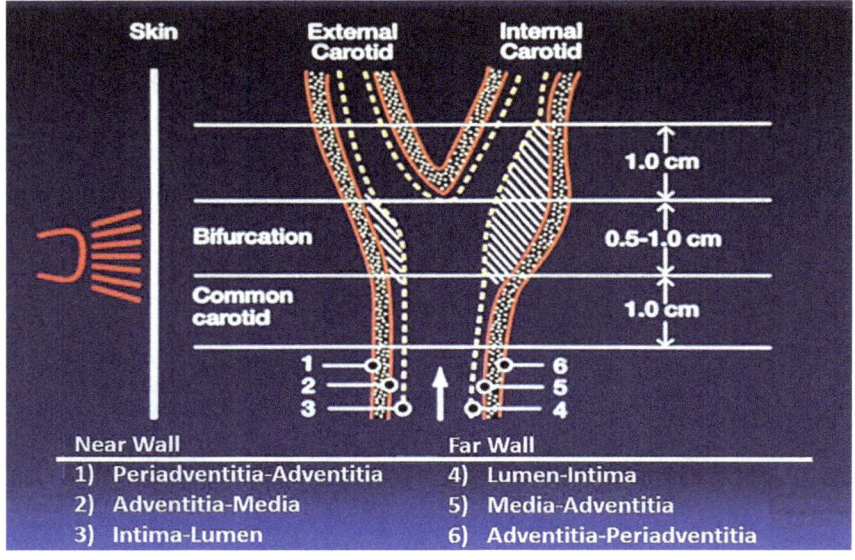

Image 41

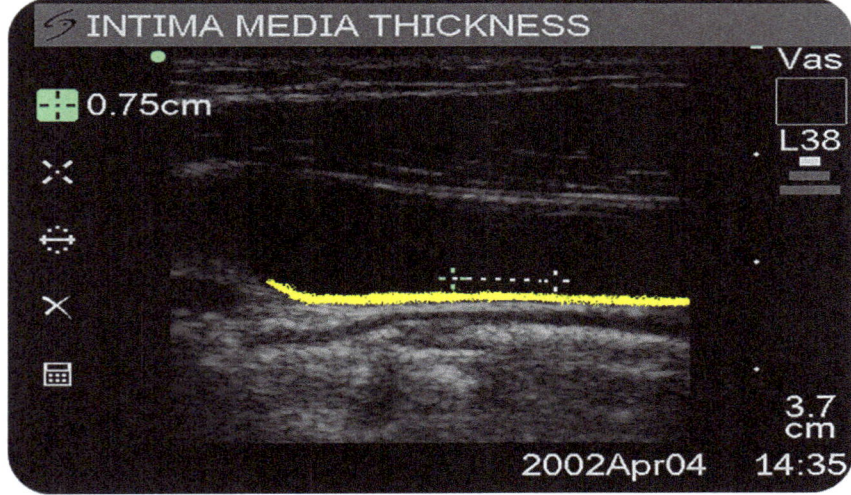

Image 42

The intima-media is the area where lipids and other pathogens and free radicals get trapped causing inflammation and launching the phagocytic cascade. It is relatively easy to image – but difficult to get reliable and reproducible measures. More on this later.

The first set of images you see below are from two different patients, one with (Image 43) and one without (Image 44) arterial inflammation. Inflammation is difficult to see with the naked eye, but I've chosen two patients' images which were taken at approximately the same depth and magnification. You should be able to detect that the inflamed artery is much thicker than that of the normal artery.

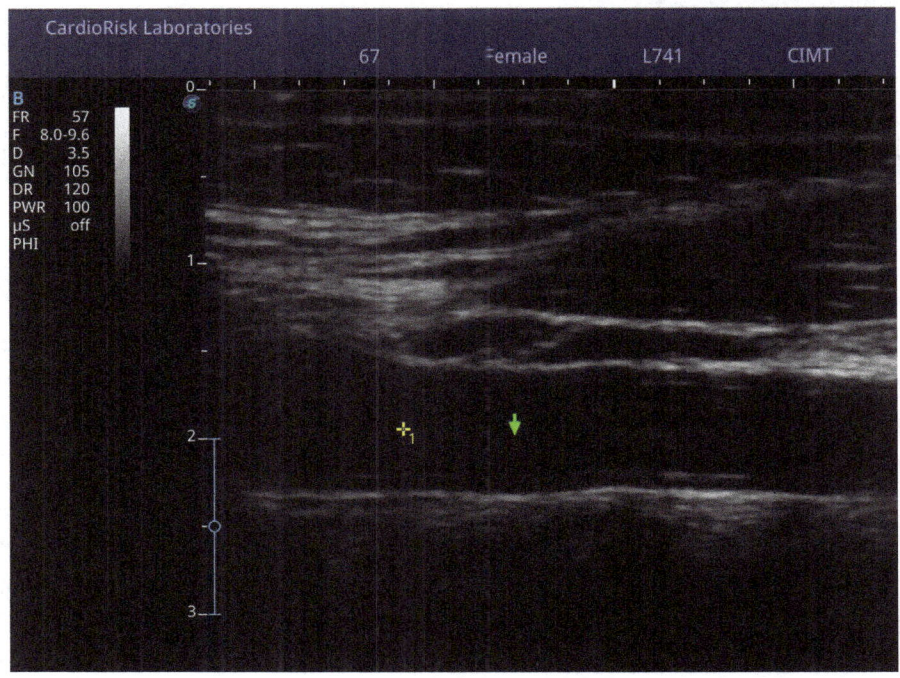

Image 43

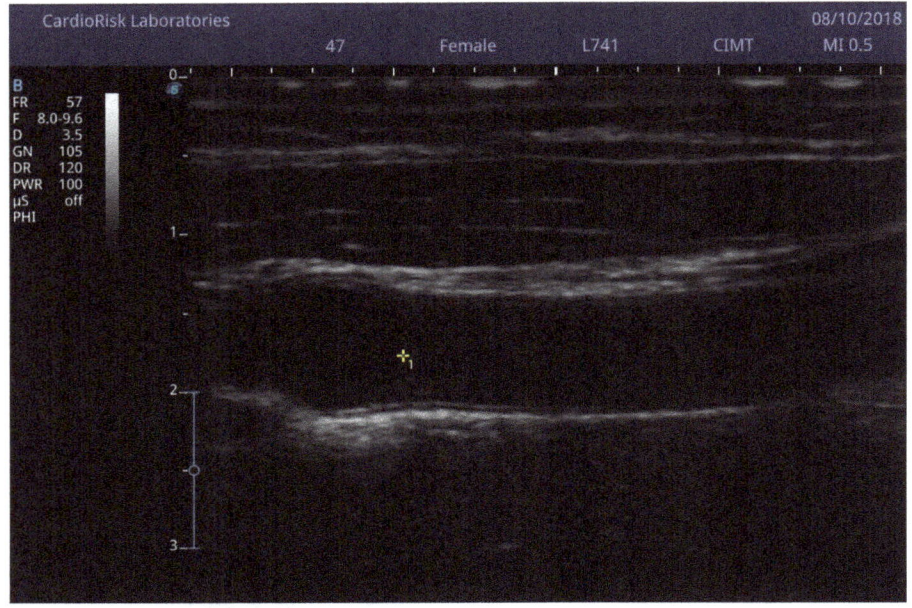

Image 44

From a technical perspective, any measurement of these two layers would qualify as an IMT measurement. However, we have already established that what and where you measure are nearly as important as whether you measure at all.

In diseased arteries, and even in pre-diseased arteries, the intima-medial wall often measures thicker the closer you take that measurement to the origin of the bifurcation. Because of the physical structure of the bifurcation in the common carotid, blood flow eddies (or circular currents of blood) are often created. These eddies allow extra time and opportunity for pathogens such as cholesterol to penetrate the arterial wall. The result of these eddies is that bifurcations often have the earliest inflammation which can be visualized by B-mode ultrasound.

Protocols which fail to establish clear anatomical markers which specifically delineate where to start and stop the IMT measurement, often experience reproducibility issues without even being aware that such a problem exists. Using the same IMT edge detection software, we tested this theory on 1000 sets of CIMT images. The result was that starting measurement acquisition at different locations proximally from the origin of the bifurcation resulted in as much as 35% variability in the measurement. The more inflamed the artery, the more variability in the measurement. It is therefore imperative that effective scanning and reading protocols acquire images from the same anatomical location and as much as possible, from the same angle. It is crucial that subsequent measurements of the interfaces are conducted from these same clearly defined anatomical markers. Failure to do so will result in unpredictable results which could lead to less than ideal treatment recommendations.

DISPARITY IN SCAN PROTOCOLS IN THE LITERATURE

Some of the confusion on CIMT stems from the fact that different scanning or imaging protocols have been used by different researchers, so the literature reveals a wide variety of disparate measuring modalities.

It would be a critical mistake to compare one study to another without first having a detailed look at the imaging methodology. For example, some studies use an average of a mean. This consists of taking several or several hundred measurements, usually from several different angles, then averaging them together and reporting their mean.

Others take a single measurement of the thickest IMT on either the right or the left carotid arteries and report that value (A Max Region). Some protocols include plaque in the average of their mean, others deliberately exclude all plaque. This results in tremendous differences between study reported results.

Even the definition of an atherosclerotic plaque varies in the literature between the most respected research laboratories. The range of plaque measurements generally vacillates between 1.0mm and 1.5mm.

A measurement of 1.5mm is nearly universally accepted as an atherosclerotic lesion in the literature, while a focal area which measures ≤ 1.0mm in nearly completely rejected as atherosclerotic plaque in the literature.

Understanding the differences in measurement technique and image acquisition protocols is imperative to interpretation of the data, the published results, and especially in comparing measurements between peer reviewed publications.

The most commonly used CIMT measure found in peer reviewed CIMT studies and included in large meta-analysis are from the far wall of the common carotid artery IMT. However, a large disparity in the number of measurements and the number of angles from which the measurements were derived exists. Disparity also exists in defining where to start and stop the measurements. Many vendors do not even define where the measurements begin and end. This should be a huge and glaring warning sign and you should stay away from vendors who have not clearly defined this.

Also – a loose definition such as "the distal 1 cm" does not adequately address the nuance of anatomical boundaries nor where the distal common carotid ends and the carotid bifurcation begins. These are crucial differentiators because the IMT tends to thicken right before the origin of the bifurcation. Using a vendor or sonographer that cannot clearly define these boundaries is almost guaranteeing variability beyond what would be acceptable or even useful in a clinical setting. The significance of these issues is discussed more at length in this book's chapter dealing with Statistics.

It's important to understand that the segments that are affected the most by the atherosclerotic process (bifurcation and internal carotid artery) were excluded in most of the meta-analysis studies that were published. It has long been known that the bifurcation and internal carotid artery develop plaque generally in advance of the common carotid artery. Another way to think about this is that the common carotid far wall IMT is predictive of plaque, and plaque is predictive of clinical events. Unfortunately, much of the known literature on this subject does not differentiate between the two methods.

Eighty percent of the intima-media thickness measured in the common carotid artery is contributed by the thickness of the muscular media layer. Notwithstanding this fact, areas of plaque were specifically excluded from most of the interventional studies. Researchers are, therefore, excluding portions of the common carotid artery that harbor atherosclerotic disease. This is tantamount to looking for a fetus via ultrasound of the breast. Maybe that is an extreme example . . . but the fact is that most atherosclerotic plaque is found by ultrasound in the bifurcation and the internal carotid arteries. It's not that plaque is never found in the distal 1cm of the common carotid . . . it is just much less common.

While taking the average mean from the far wall of the distal 1cm in the common carotid makes sense methodologically in large intervention trials, in clinical practice we simply cannot afford to stop there. When looking for evidence of disease, which could lead to a clinical event, the presence of any plaque in any vascular segment indicates atherosclerosis and would be a critical finding. The CAFES-CAVE study found that 30% of the patients with normal carotid arteries had femoral arteriosclerotic lesions (Belcaro, 2001). Looking beyond the distal 1cm of the common carotid is critical to a comprehensive exam.

Still, disparate protocols are used throughout the randomized clinical trials included in the most cited meta-analysis on IMT. For instance, in the ACAPS trial, the mean-max from 12 segments is used (Furberg, 1994). In the ASAP trial, only the far wall CCA was used (Smilde, 2001). While some researchers attempt to analyze all three segments, most simply report far wall common carotid IMT. This creates disparity and confusion in those less familiar with the method.

For example, in two landmark studies, the Rotterdam (Bots, 1997) and the Cardiovascular Health Studies (Fried, 1991), the magnitude of association with cardiovascular disease was stronger using the mean maximum CIMT estimate than it was with the common average of the mean CIMT estimate.

Another study, the Muscatine Study (Lauer, 1988), conducted in much younger subjects aged 33 to 42 years, found that the use of mean maximum IMT provided more correlations (9 versus 0) and more significant correlations (p 0.05 [26 versus 19] and p 0.001 [14 versus 1]) with current risk factor levels than with the use of only common carotid artery measurements of CIMT.

Researchers should be extremely clear and perhaps even obsessive at designing their protocols not just to monitor inflammation (a process most easily tracked by monitoring the far wall of the distal 1cm in the common carotid) but also in tracking active atherosclerotic disease (a process most effectively tracked by looking for focal atherosclerotic lesions in as many arterial segments as can be visualized, and by looking for them on both the near and far walls, and from as many angles as patient anatomy will allow). Clinicians need to be aware of the difference and insist their IMT provider has clearly defined protocols which will assess the arteries using both methods. Only then will comparison between studies yield meaningful results relating to comparative findings.

PLAQUE – THE SILENT KILLER AND THE MISSING VARIABLE IN MUCH OF THE LITERATURE

Meta-analysis research published in the JACC (Costanzo, 2010) and AHJ (Lorenz M. B., 2010) do not take into consideration changes in plaque area or calcification. These changes are not only clinically relevant, but they speak more to the probability of future events.

The mean common carotid IMT is easier to track and is an important biomarker to monitor inflammation – but you will not see additional change in the mean common carotid IMT in a patient who has been treated therapeutically for many years. Never was this more true than in the Enhance trial (Kastelein, 2005). To refresh your memory, the Ezetimibe enhanced arm of this trial showed a slight progression not regression of mean IMT.

There were multiple factors that contributed to the seemingly confounding nature of this trial's results. For starters, the beginning mean IMT values were significantly different between the two groups – one managed to normal at 0.695mm and the other average exceeded the upper 75% percentile for risk.

Add to this the fact that many of the patients in the Ezetimibe leg had already undergone aggressive statin therapy for a number of years so that whatever inflammation they may have once had in the walls of their arteries, had long since been corrected. For these reasons and many others, it is important we look at both mean IMT, Max Region IMT, and that any clinical exam include a comprehensive assessment of plaque in as many vascular beds as is feasible.

Monitoring the presence of plaque then, and the relative echogenicity of these lesions as presented in grey scale densitometry is vital to monitoring active disease progression. The pathophysiology of this disease is such that inflammation leads to plaque formation.

Initially plaques are soft, and densitometrically echoluscent, and extremely vulnerable to rupture. Echoluscency refers to the sound wave signature as reflected on the screen. Sound waves bounce off different material at different rates. These are then presented to an ultrasound screen in brightness mode (b-mode) such that the dark colors are the signature of less dense . . . even liquid form material, while bright white colors are the signature of intensely dense material.

As this disease progresses, minerals such as calcium are attracted to the lesion to help stabilize and heal the wound. The presence of increased calcium in the plaque lesion is visualized by more bright white sound signals. The bright white on a plaque is visual evidence of calcium and other minerals which are a signal that the lesion is healing. The more bright white that can be seen on the image, the more stable it is and the less vulnerable to rupture it will be.

Another way to think about this is with regards to facial acne. Most of us could feel an acne lesion forming on our face long before we could see redness on the epidermis of our skin. We knew a lesion was imminent because we could feel it. It was often painful to touch. The pain was caused by nerve receptors which were activated by the subdermal inflammation just beneath the skin's surface. Left untreated, a small white head pimple could eventually be seen visibly in a mirror, along with a slightly reddish circle surrounding the lesion (inflammation plus disease).

If that lesion did not rupture, it would continue its evolution and the soft white material inside the lesion would eventually fill with a cottage cheese looking substance. That substance is necrotic material left over from the phagocytic process. This cottage cheese looking substance is already much more difficult to rupture than its softer and more liquid-like predecessor. Because of its thicker consistency, these lesions often grow in size.

Once again, if the lesion does not rupture, it would eventually form a hard ball of material very much like a cyst just beneath the surface of the skin. This final phase of disease progression often requires a surgical removal (either by a trained or untrained professional) because it is now extremely resistant to rupture.

Plaque is metaphorically and pathophysiologically very similar to that of acne. The underlying phagocytic disease process is very similar. This is why some of the other structural wall imaging technologies occasionally miss patients with active disease.

A Coronary Artery Calcium Score (CACC), for example, is an extremely attractive modality which successfully identifies patients at risk for future events. However – one of its weaknesses is that it scores the calcified plaque, not the soft, echoluscent plaque which is most vulnerable to rupture. Remember that calcium build up on a plaque lesion is a final phase of the disease.

Don't get me wrong, CACC scan are still extremely important. They provide a better view into the coronary arteries. They also do a phenomenal job at flagging patients at need for immediate surgical intervention – but they do not 'see' soft and vulnerable plaque as readily.

Let's get back to plaque. Understanding that basic pathophysiology is vital to understanding the relevance of a properly performed IMT exam which looks at both monitorable inflammation, but also plaque or active atherosclerotic disease presence and more importantly, plaque rupture vulnerability.

Another study found that there were seven times the number of total coronary events in patients with vulnerable soft plaque than in those without it (Honda, 2004). There were 9.5 times as many patients with ACS in the patients who had vulnerable plaque than in those without it.

This underscores the fact that while all plaque is dangerous, no matter the size, some plaque (vulnerable, soft, & echoluscent) are many times more dangerous than their echogenic cousins. Care needs to be taken to make sure that your IMT vendor understands the difference, and more importantly, that they have a detailed protocol in place to correctly identify and report the difference.

As relating to IMT literature, the main underlying problem is that missing plaque data and the separation between plaque identification and inflammatory monitoring will almost always lead to bias in the CIMT progression rates and the published results or interpretation of data. Imagine conducting a pregnancy trial where you eliminated all women with big bellies. You might still find some pregnant women, but you would miss far too many. This is what happened in many of the IMT intervention trials – plaque (a direct measure of atherosclerotic disease) was deliberately removed from the study.

It should be stated that the **best** protocols are those that look at <u>both</u> the mean maximum CIMT and the average mean CIMT, along with a comprehensive interrogation of each arterial segment bilaterally for plaque. The protocols then need to characterize each plaque for echogenicity and vulnerability. Together this set of criteria create the optimal CIMT assessment protocol.

B-mode ultrasound images of plaque are crucial to effective risk management and prescriptive therapy. The images below show patients with plaque. Each of these patients are in need of aggressive pharmacological therapy regardless of their blood or functional test results.

Image 45, shows a 49 year old patient whose only other immediately identifiable risks for heart attack and stroke included family history. An uncle experienced an MI while in his late 60's. This is not a patient that most physicians would get too excited about treating aggressively right away.

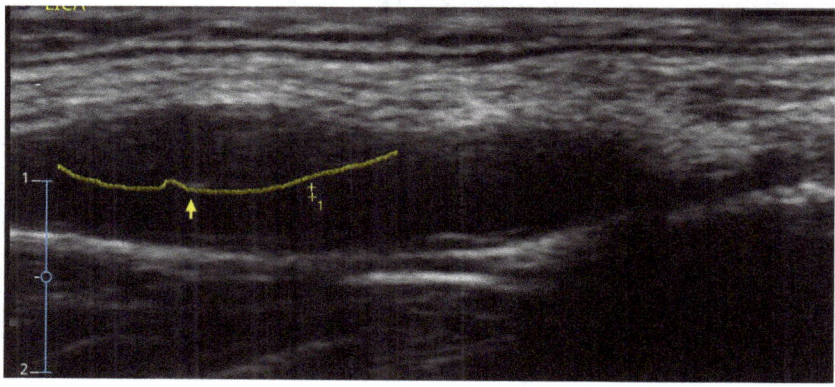

Image 45

In the patient's transverse plane image shown in Image 46, we can see that the patient is nowhere near meeting the criteria for a surgical intervention (e.g. he is <70% occluded and asymptomatic). Even though a full duplex exam may need to be considered, we can see that this patient's occlusion does not quite approach even a 50% occlusion.

Should we be worried? YES! Absolutely! Statistically, this patient has the same risk of having a cardio or cerebrovascular event as someone who has already had one (Johnsen, 2007). How would knowing this information change the way you approach this patient's therapeutic recommendations? If you look closely, you can see that it is echolucent – heterogenous. There is no echoic shadow or fallout which you would see in a completely echogenic lesion. Also, notice that the color signature of black in some portions of this plaque are black = liquid = the same ultrasound signature as blood. Only the slightest shades of bright white speckle appear in the longitudinal plane. This patient's lesion is vulnerable to rupture. Wouldn't it make sense to try to stabilize the lesion so that it does not erupt or erode and cause trauma?

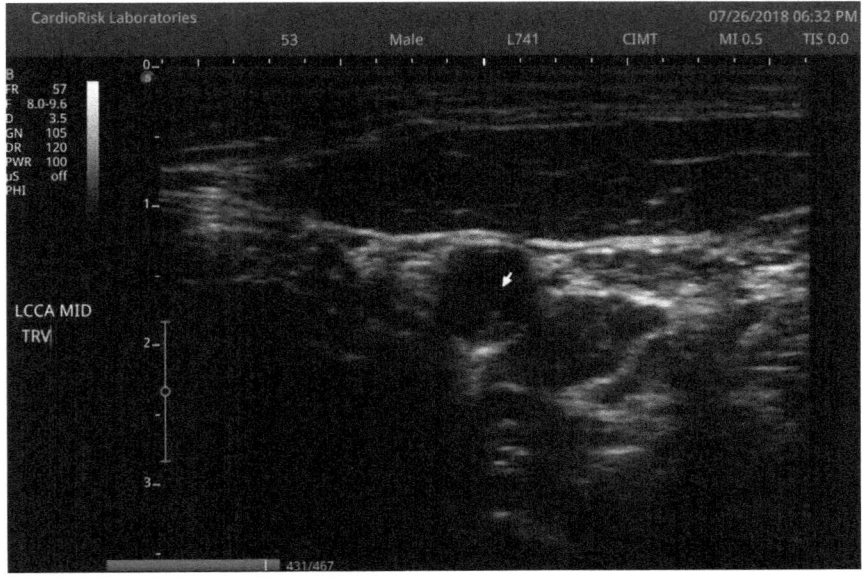

Image 46

The patient whose artery we see in Image 47 is also relatively young (53 years at the time of imaging). I've outlined his soft plaque so that you can get a flavor for its mass, its echolucency and its vulnerability. This plaque is roughly four inches from this patients' brain. Wouldn't you be concerned if this were your patient?

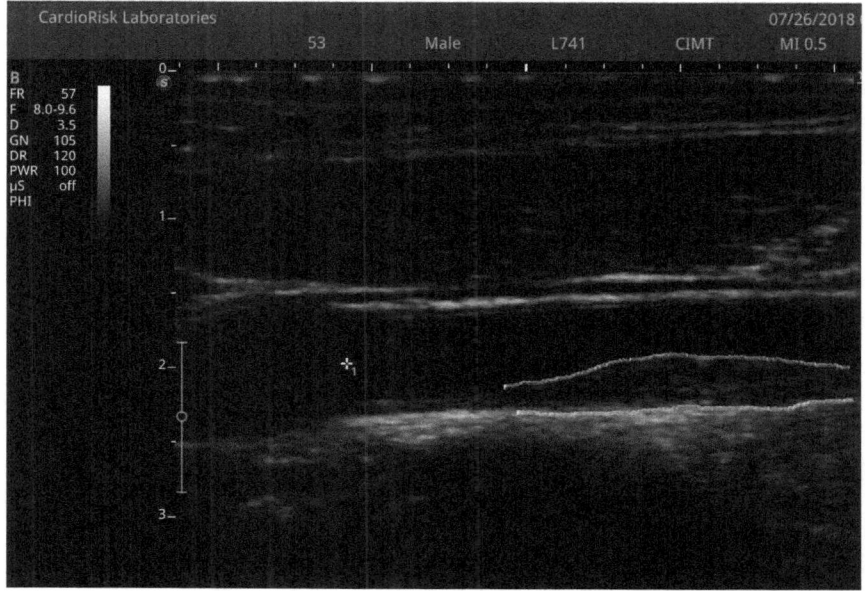

Image 47

The combination of Average Mean, Max Region, the interrogation of as many vascular beds as is prudent for plaque, and then the densitometric evaluation of that plaque for rupture vulnerability will add significant information to your ability to identify those patients at need for aggressive therapy. Monitoring these conditions over time is extremely useful to assess whether or not your prescriptive advice is having the intended health outcome on your patients. If you haven't already, I urge you to begin using IMT in your practice right now!

MISUNDERSTOOD INTERPRETATION OF THE META-ANALYSIS – AKA:THE 'NAY SAYERS'.

"If we are to have credibility in the scientific community then we must embrace not just that which supports our views and beliefs, but we must also look deeply into that science which may contradict our beliefs. Only after we have delved deeply into the data which supports and contrasts our own thoughts and beliefs can we be sure we have been intellectually honest in our pursuit of truth."

- TODD ELDREDGE 2012

CONTROVERSY IN THE META-ANALYSIS TREATING INDIVIDUALIZED DISEASE

Numerous methods exist to stratify risk in a patient: The Framingham risk score, LDL, CRP, Lp(a), etc. Notwithstanding these methods to assess risk in the individual patient, there is currently no standard means of assessing benefit to the individual patient. Improving LDL, blood pressure, or CRP does not assure that the underlying atherosclerotic process has been slowed or halted in that particular patient.

It is sobering to realize that data from a 2008 study revealed that nearly 75% of over 137,000 patients admitted to the hospital with CAD had LDL levels below 130 mg/dL and nearly 50% had LDL levels below 100 mg/dL (Sachdeva A. C., 2009). So, how ethical is it to tell your patient that "all is well" because their LDL is less than100mg/dL, when half of those admitted to the hospital with an ischemic event have achieved a "desirable" LDL level of <100 mg/dL?

The truth is that it is currently nearly impossible to know how much intervention is needed to halt the atherosclerotic process in an individual patient. Lowering an LDL to under 70 in a high-risk individual still leaves residual risk in some patients, but in which ones?

The use of serial CIMT monitoring would allow the customization of treatment to the individual. Individualized medicine is the future. After all, if one had a tool to prove atherosclerosis was regressing in an individual patient this would be of enormous clinical significance.

Multiple individual studies have shown the predictive value of serial CIMT measurements to monitor efficacy of treatment. Yet, one large meta-analysis did not support this concept and another one supports it, but only marginally.

It is not surprising that the benefit of serial monitoring is not evident in these studies considering the disparity between different protocols used in the dozens of studies pooled, the lack of multiple segment analysis, variability in excess of the change being measured, many without any statements concerning reproducibility, and most with no plaque analysis, all with disparate interventions and disparate inclusion criteria.

PRECEDENTS IN MEDICINE

A well-known and acceptable medical practice uses change in tumor size on CT scanning to assess benefit of chemotherapy or radiation. This is done without the benefit of randomized, placebo-controlled intervention trials.

Should serial monitoring of CIMT be condemned because the definitive intervention trial has not or may never be performed? Of course not, that would be nonsense.

Espeland, et al. stated that CIMT meets Prentice's criteria to serve as a surrogate biomarker for cardiovascular disease endpoints in statin trials (Espeland, 2005). This conclusion was reached, notwithstanding the fact that it was based on a meta-analysis of different published CIMT studies, each using a different imaging and reading protocol.

Still, others continue to attempt to minimize CIMT's utility as a surrogate endpoint for disease or even as a useful clinical tool because it does not, yet, have a randomized, placebo-controlled intervention trial.

There are very real difficulties with obtaining reproducible CIMT scans. Yet, a peer-reviewed publication of the CardioRisk protocol demonstrates that with proper training of technician and readers, variability of CIMT scan results of the same patient can be managed to a range of 0.002 mm in arithmetic variability, with a standard deviation of 0.02mm (Riches, 2010). You would be hard pressed to find another test in any genre of medicine with tighter coefficients of variability. Certainly, this degree of reproducibility increases the usefulness of serial CIMT monitoring in clinical practice. It was not, however, available in most of the studies considered in the two meta-analysis which were less favorable on the method.

Plaque measurement represents its own set of obstacles where even slight changes in the angle of the transducer can lead to much larger changes in the resulting measurements. These conditions contribute to a lower reproducibility of plaque measurement and make it much more difficult for meaningful tracking of a single plaque lesion than it is to track the average mean of several hundred measurements in the distal common carotid.

A study by CardioRisk (Riches, 2010) showed that plaque reproducibility can be managed effectively through the use of a defined protocol, and via the certification and training of all operators. Another study noted that plaques provide great clinical benefit in proving efficacy of treatment by simply counting the number of plaques and by adding the plaque volume as measured by three-dimensional volumetric reporting (Landry, 2005). Perhaps an exact measurement of plaque is less important than other factors.

DOES SERIAL MONITORING OF CIMT PREDICT RISK?

Several large epidemiologic studies: ARIC (Chambless, 1997) (Chambless, 2000), CHS (O'Leary, 1992), Rotterdam (Bots, 1997), & CAPS (Lorenz M. V., 2005)) demonstrate that a baseline measurement of the intima-media thickness of the common carotid artery (CIMT) correlates strongly with risk for myocardial infarction and cerebrovascular events.

Recommendations to consider including a baseline CIMT in the assessment of an individual patient have surfaced both in the United States and Europe. (European Society of Hypertension–European Society of Cardiology (Mancia, 2013), American Heart Association (Greenland, 2000)).

The Framingham risk score (based on examination, history and laboratory evaluation) has been used for many years with wide acceptance to determine risk in the individual patient. Adding a baseline CIMT to a Framingham risk score to further stratify the individual patient has also gained acceptance.

All humans are born with a surprisingly uniform IMT of the common carotid (CIMT) of 0.4mm. The landmark China study showed that thickening of the arteries does not appear to be related to age (Campbell, 2004). However, that population had no risk factors.

In a US population it is theoretically impossible to find a cohort without any risk factors. Environmental, eating choices, and other lifestyle choices make some risks nearly impossible to avoid. Indeed, in persons in the United States with no known traditional risk factors, CIMT thickness does appear to increase with age, to approximately 0.8mm by the age of 80 (Chambless, 1997). It is the deviation from this expected slope that accounts for the observation in epidemiologic trials and which allows CIMT to be used to assess risk.

So the question on the table is: Does serial scanning provide additional benefit?

It has long been assumed that changes between successive CIMT measurements would reflect a change in this slope and could therefore reflect an increase or decrease in risk from what was expected. In other words, not only could the baseline CIMT be used for initial risk stratification, but the change that may occur between successive scans could be used to refine risk even further and to measure efficacy of treatment (Naqvi, 2014). Numerous intervention trials have been carried out on this premise. Progression or regression of CIMT has been equated to failure or success of lifestyle, dietary, or pharmaceutical interventions.

In the METEOR trial (Crouse, 2007), the FDA used the observation that rosuvastatin caused a decrease in the expected progression of CIMT as measured between serial scans to award an additional indication in their package insert: Slowing the progression of atherosclerosis served as part of a treatment strategy to lower total-C and LDL-C in addition to diet.

The FDA granted a new indication for rosuvastatin based solely on the CIMT change rate. If CIMT serial monitoring was good enough for the FDA . . . why would it be any less applicable for patients in your practice?

A look at the ARBITER trial reveals a similar assessment (Taylor, 2006). The treated patient cohort experienced a net regression of 0.027mm (± 0.011mm – p<0.001 vs. placebo). Although extended release niacin has had its share of issues, once again we see the FDA acting on the results of a trial where CIMT was the primary clinical endpoint.

In the METEOR (Crouse, 2007) and ARBITER (Taylor, 2006) trials, and in virtually every other intervention trial involving CIMT conducted in the United States, absolute CIMT is not taken into consideration in the final assessment of clinical efficacy of treatment. What is taken into consideration is the *amount of change* that has occurred between scans.

It is often stated that the Food and Drug Administration has recognized CIMT as a surrogate marker for cardiovascular events. More precisely, the FDA recognizes that "The CIMT change rate" is a surrogate marker for cardiovascular events.

The American Heart Journal published another meta-analysis that looked at 28 randomized controlled intervention trials that measured serial changes in CIMT and compared them to clinical outcomes (Goldberger, 2010). This comprehensive meta-analysis published in the American Heart Journal in 2010 found that less progression in CIMT over time was associated with a lower likelihood of non-fatal MI. However, the authors concluded, "Less progression in CIMT over time is associated with a lower likelihood of nonfatal MI in selected randomized controlled trials; however, these findings were inconsistent at times, suggesting caution in using CIMT as a surrogate end point."

The conclusions reached by these meta-analyses have caused much discussion among researchers and clinicians. We have already addressed some of the problems that exist in attempting to reach conclusive results when comparing studies which use different image acquisition protocols. One of the many weaknesses of this particular study is the wide variety of studies chosen to evaluate the efficacy of the modality.

MANAGING THE INDIVIDUAL PATIENT

The ultimate goal is to apply CIMT findings to the management of the individual patient. Baseline risk stratification by a single CIMT measurement requires less reproducibility than comparing the relatively small change between successive scans in the same patient.

As the trials analyzed in the two meta-analyses (AHJ (Goldberger, 2010) and JACC (Costanzo, 2010) used a variety of scan protocols, a variety of older and newer technologies, and because the reproducibility was often unstated, it is not surprising the general impression in these two publications, was that change over time was poorly correlated with outcomes.

Without careful attention to the details of transducer angulation, the area being measured, gain settings, certification of readers and sonographers, and other quality control and quality assurance measures to ensure reproducibility, the conclusions reached concerning serial monitoring are not surprising. Garbage in = Garbage out.

In the peer-reviewed study with CardioRisk sonographers and readers, the reproducibility of a common carotid mean IMT in an office setting for an individual patient is readily achieved at 0.002mm arithmetically with a standard deviation of 0.02mm (Riches, 2010). This level of quality and reproducibility was clearly not demonstrated in the studies referenced by either of these two meta-analyses.

The degree of accuracy and reproducibility must be taken into consideration as researchers and clinicians consider using serial monitoring to determine efficacy of treatment. If the measured change between scans is greater than the error of the method, then the clinician can be certain a change has taken place. However, the clinician must be aware of the error of the method before conclusions can be drawn that the change measured is real, and not a reflection of the error of the measurement.

CHANGE OVER TIME IS A SURROGATE FOR CLINICAL EVENTS

The AHJ and JACC meta-analyses include trials that examined a variety of different interventions. It has been concluded previously by Espeland, O'Leary and others regarding statin intervention trials (through a meta-analysis of 7 such trials) that *change in CIMT meets accepted criteria as a surrogate for clinical events* (Espeland, 2005).

Based on their meta-analysis with both CIMT and clinical event outcomes, statin therapy was associated with an average reduction in CIMT of .012mm/yr. compared with placebo. Also, these trials showed that there was a significant reduction in the odds ratio for a cardiovascular event in patients receiving statin therapy.

The meta-analysis in JACC included 41 intervention trials, 21 of which were statin trials. The conclusions drawn from the meta-analysis of Espeland and O'Leary are in conflict with that of the JACC meta-analysis, yet both included either exclusively or largely statin trials in their analysis.

WHO IS SCANNING, WHO IS READING, AND WHO IS CERTIFYING? THE CRUCIAL DIFFERENCE.

An analysis from the European Lacidipine Study on Atherosclerosis (ELSA) Study, a multicenter (23 sites, 50 sonographers, 9 readers) randomized clinical trial, showed the highest intraclass correlation coefficient (0.89) when the sonographer and the reader were the same at both visits (Zanchetti, 1998). This would be achievable in an office setting but is not achievable in a meta-analysis that included randomized clinical trials that absolutely used different sonographers and readers.

Several years ago, I attended a CIMT training for a group of physicians at a trade meeting for the detection and treatment of atherosclerosis. In this meeting, the group of 75 or so physicians were learning how to read (how to measure the IMT) using the latest edge detection software. All participants used the exact same set of images so that there was zero variation between the scan images.

After 3 days of training with the software, the closest that any two physicians in the group came to the measurements of any other physician was 0.10mm. Now think about that in the context of what we know about standard deviation (more on this in the chapter on Statistics). This would mean that were it even possible to eliminate ALL variability from the acquired and saved images of a patient, using standardized edge detection software, this group would be unable to detect a change in the IMT of their patients with a $\geq 95\%$ confidence if that change was < 0.20mm. A measurement of 0.30mm is approximately 1/3 of the total size of the measurement of an at-risk artery in the upper tertile of risk. Unfortunately, this much variability would be completely unacceptable in clinical practice since the difference between a healthy and an unhealthy artery in the ARIC study was in the neighborhood of 0.08mm (Chambless, 1997). This should give us pause before selecting a CIMT vendor who has not undergone both training and double-blind performance-based certification by an independent 3rd party.

DIFFERENT STUDY GROUPS, DIFFERENT SCAN PROTOCOLS, DIFFERENT RATES OF CHANGE, & DIFFERENT INTERVENTIONS = DIFFERENT RESULTS

Does the lack of correlation of outcomes with changes which were observed in pharmaceutical trials reflect the deleterious effects of medication that might blunt the expected benefits one would expect from a change in CIMT? Conversely, are there off-target benefits in terms of events that might confound the expected results based on CIMT alone? What if a meta-analysis was done of non-pharmaceutical interventions alone? Is there another way to look at the data that would allow the clinician to attach special importance to the change between successive scans?

Analysis of existing data is difficult. CIMT as a technology is suffering in part from its own successes. As technological advances are made, and scan protocols are improved, each study is different from the previous one. This makes direct comparisons between studies difficult (just as in drug therapeutic trials).

For instance, earlier studies cited in both of these meta-analysis, commonly relied on the analysis of a minimum of measurements from at least 2 images obtained from ultrasound transducers which featured 7-10 megahertz. The Arbiter trials used 6, 8, and 16 image measurements which were obtained using ultrasound transducers set to 13MHz (Taylor, 2006). This further complicates and confounds comparisons between earlier and later studies.

While a vast amount of data can be gathered by performing B-mode ultrasound interrogation of the extracranial carotid artery, its predictive power will depend largely on what exactly is measured, how accurately it is measured and how often it is measured.

The internal carotid artery, the bifurcation of the common and common carotid artery all contain information of potential clinical use. As technology evolves it is evident that an integration of information gathered from all areas is necessary to optimize the predictive power of the measurements. This new data will be very difficult to compare to the technologies and scanning protocols from prior studies.

CORRELATION BETWEEN CIMT AND CORONARY ANGIOGRAPHY

There is a significant relationship between progression of coronary artery disease as assessed by the change in percent diameter stenosis using quantitative coronary angiography and coronary events (Azen, 1996). Serial coronary angiography in an individual patient would therefore be useful in predicting the likelihood of future coronary events in that patient. Not degree of stenosis, but the *change* in stenosis between successive angiographies.

Due to the invasive nature of coronary angiography, the potential exposure or overexposure to radiation, and the inconvenience to the patient, assessing future risk by coronary angiography is impractical for managing atherosclerosis in the majority of patients. It also is not warranted in the primary prevention of cardiovascular disease. Coronary angiography is really a study of lumenography or a look into the amount or percent blockage of the lumen.

As we've already discussed, the atherosclerotic process often begins in the intima-media layers of the coronary artery, causing an expansion of these layers. This expansion occurs outwardly and inwardly. The expansion outwardly occurs in advance of the inward expansion towards the lumen or blood flow, leading to significant thickening of the intima-media layer long before any encroachment upon the lumen. Lumenography assesses the end-stage process of atherosclerosis – or the actual clogging or stenosis of the vessel.

The intima-media must become thickened before the coronary artery lumen becomes narrowed. Heart attacks can occur in blood vessels in which the stenosis is less than 50%. This happens due to sudden plaque rupture often followed by clot formation at the site of rupture. In fact, this appears to be the case in over 65% of heart attacks (Falk, 1995). A subject who has a coronary angiogram showing 50% or less stenosis is still at significant risk for acute myocardial infarction as over half of the events studied occurred in people with less than 50% stenosis.

Measurement of the intima-media thickness, which is independent of degree of stenosis, would have revealed changes in advance of stenosis of the arterial lumen. There is a strong association between the thickness of the intima-media layer and stenosis of the arterial lumen. Assessment of the intima-media thickness by ultrasonography has been shown to be a useful surrogate for coronary angiography with correlations exceeding 90% (Coskun, 2009).

A logical next step would be for the office-based physician to utilize CIMT as a surrogate for coronary angiography to assess progression of coronary artery disease and coronary events. Critics have stated the reproducibility of IMT measurements is too poor to be utilized in the individual patient. Critics also cite the fact that no carefully-designed prospective study has been performed to prove or disprove the assertion that intima-media ultrasonography can be used to follow the progression of coronary artery disease. The aforementioned meta-analyses will be used by critics to support their position.

LESSONS FROM INDIVIDUAL RANDOMIZED CLINICAL TRIALS

While meta-analyses can help draw conclusions that are not obtainable from review of single studies, it is useful to examine individual studies that reach different conclusions than the meta-analysis itself. I have included four of these studies below for your review. Be aware that some of these studies were included in the metanalyses described above.

The first two studies which were designed specifically to address the contribution of change over time to risk stratification were CLAS (Blankenhorn, 1987) and Carotid Plaque Area (Spence, 2002).

CLAS compared baseline intima-media thickness in two study groups: 1) a low cholesterol diet plus colestipol and niacin 2) a low cholesterol diet plus placebo. In CLAS, the *rate of change* of pre-intrusive carotid atherosclerosis determined by measurement of the intima-media thickness of the distal common carotid arterial far wall **was** predictive of coronary events.

For each 0.03mm increase per year in common carotid arterial intima-media thickness, the relative risk for nonfatal myocardial infarction or coronary death was 2.2, and the relative risk for nonfatal myocardial infarction, coronary death, or a revascularization procedure was 3.1. This is a significant finding which is absolutely applicable in the private physician setting.

This relationship with coronary events was similar in the placebo group and the drug group; in addition, the absolute measurement of the intima-media thickness of the distal common carotid artery far wall was predictive of coronary events. It is significant to note that after adjustment for the intima media thickness change rate, the effect of treatment on nonfatal myocardial infarction or coronary death was no longer apparent. This finding indicates that the measurement of the intima-media thickness change rate was mediated by the effect of treatment on coronary events (Blankenhorn, 1987).

Many risk factors that contribute to the progression of atherosclerosis are shared by the two arterial beds (Persson, 1994). In CLAS, it was shown that carotid arterial intima-media thickness incorporates additional, independent information on prediction of coronary events beyond the angiographic measurement of luminal narrowing mechanism. That is, a minimal improvement in lumen diameter is associated with a marked decrease in coronary events. This is probably based on the increase in lumen size being a reflection of plaque stabilization and/or decrease in intima-media thickness either of which signify a significant decrease in the likelihood of future cardiac events.

One could imply from the data presented in CLAS that the measurement of the intima-media thickness change rate was mediated by the effect of treatment on coronary events over time, and even more so than by the absolute thickness of the CIMT as measured at any one point in time. This might be construed as evidence that once a coronary event has occurred or once one has determined that severe atherosclerosis exists in a patient, that using the absolute thickness of a carotid intima-media measurement in isolation loses its predictive value. This could be because these patients are already at such high risk from plaque deposition that a simple measurement of the intima-media thickness of the common carotid artery is simply not as predictive of future events, whereas the change in absolute thickness in the treated group was predictive of future events. Measuring change in the arterial wall, particularly that change found in the average of the mean in the common carotid, is a direct measure of inflammation. When inflammation is active, disease is active. There is only one place for an inflamed artery to go and that is the formation of atherosclerotic plaques. Conversely, reduction of the amount of inflammation in the wall of the artery, reflects the efficacy of disease management whether that management be in the form of pharmaceuticals or mere lifestyle modification.

This would make serial measurements, which monitor inflammation in the wall of the artery, of extreme importance in persons who have had coronary stents, bypass grafting, acute coronary syndrome or prior MI. In the CLAS study, the outcomes in the treated group were significantly improved over the untreated group (Blankenhorn, 1987).

In addition, after adjustment for the intima-media thickness change rate, the effect of treatment on nonfatal myocardial infarction or coronary death was no longer apparent. This finding would indicate that the measurement of the intima-media thickness change rate was mediated through the effect of treatment on coronary events.

Still, no sub-analysis was performed where comparisons were made in the treated group of patients between those showing regression and those showing progression of intima media thickness. The CLAS article concludes by saying, "To the extent that common carotid arterial intima-media thickness progression is associated with risk of coronary events, a potentially enormous clinical significance is linked to the noninvasive assessment of the progression of early pre-intrusive atherosclerosis."

In Carotid Plaque Area (Spence, 2002), Spence, et al, looked specifically at the rate of change of plaque area and found the correlation of this change with degree of risk.

It is important to note that in this study, those showing progression of plaque had the most events. The burden of atherosclerosis could be measured as total carotid plaque area using two-dimensional ultrasound; and this quantity was a strong predictor of cardiovascular outcomes. Patients in the top quartile of carotid plaque had 3.4 times the risk of stroke, death or myocardial infarction over 5 years compared to patients in the lowest quartile, even after adjustment for age, sex, cholesterol, systolic blood pressure, smoking, diabetes, homocysteine, and treatment of lipids and blood pressure.

Patients with plaque progression, despite treatment of traditional risk factors, have twice the risk as those with stable plaque or regression even after adjustment for the same risk factors.

Plaque is biologically and genetically distinct from intima–media thickness, stenosis, and other phenotypes of atherosclerosis such as coronary calcium. Plaque area was more sensitive and specific for identifying patients free of coronary artery stenosis than were the average mean IMT or coronary calcium scoring.

A third study, ELSA, followed subjects over a four-year period (Giuseppe, 2001). The ELSA study did serial CIMT (Mean Max. Measurements) and plaque analysis and then correlated these findings with events. The conclusions of this single study were more in agreement with the adverse findings of the JACC and AHJ meta-analyses, but further comment seems warranted.

Of interest is the fact that the two anti-hypertensives (lacidipine and atenolol), caused different CIMT changes over time, despite lowering blood pressure at similar rates. Lacidipine slowed progression more than Atenolol. But the outcomes for these two anti-hypertensives were not reported separately.

Atenolol has been shown in some studies to be an inferior anti-hypertensive in terms of outcomes compared to other agents, despite similar blood pressure lowering capabilities. It is conceivable that the slowing of progression was achieved in the Atenolol arm yet an increase in events occurred by some non-atherosclerosis process that led to a subsequent cardiovascular event.

A major limitation and extremely important observation of the present ELSA analysis is that patients included in this analysis were, overall, at relatively low risk. They had their hypertension well controlled by treatment. Consequently, the incidence of cardiovascular outcomes during the 4-year study was rather low. Because of this, the power of detecting correlation with an organ-specific event, such as stroke, was low. The most valuable information was derived from pooling major and minor cardiovascular outcomes, including clinically relevant events such as: hospitalized heart failure, angina, atrial fibrillation, and claudication, in addition to stroke, myocardial infarction, and cardiovascular death. This led the authors to this conclusion: "Therefore, the conclusion that carotid IMT is a significantly important added risk factor throughout long-term antihypertensive treatment appears to be particularly solid."

There were only 25 strokes in this study. This could possibly stem from the fact that patients with very thick carotid walls (e.g. IMT > 4.0 mm or those most likely to develop ischemic cerebrovascular events) **were excluded** according to the ELSA protocol. The rationale was that these lesions are unlikely to be significantly modified by treatment – so they were omitted.

It is interesting to note, once again, those patients with the highest likelihood of an event were not only excluded from this study but plaques in general were not included in the two most important meta-analyses. This undermines the validity and utility of these two meta-analysis which were used to diminish CIMT's usefulness in serial monitoring of disease.

CIMT (Mean Max) maintained its predictive value during 4 years of anti-hypertensive treatment in the ELSA study (Peters, 2013). Plaque correlated well with cardiovascular events. Serial changes in CIMT did not correlate with outcomes, yet two treatment arms with different effects on changes in CIMT were lumped together, which clearly confounds the analysis.

CLAS (Azen, 1996) and Carotid Plaque Area (Spence, 2002) were reviewed to show that two of the largest studies that were designed to assess the benefit of serial monitoring concluded in favor of the concept.

ELSA (Zanchetti, 1998) was designed to show retention of the predictive nature of a CIMT scan while on anti-hypertensive treatment. This was shown. Notwithstanding the several problems with the study cited above, the authors conclude, "These negative conclusions should be tempered by the limitations inherent in the smallness of these changes compared with the large individual differences in baseline IMTs."

Applying conclusions drawn from intervention studies of groups of patients to the individual patient is complex. Groups of patients showing regression, for instance, are really a heterogeneous group, some showing regression, and some possibly showing progression. Lumping both responders and non-responders into the same group blunts the ability to isolate out those who have significant change greater than the error of the method and assign an event rate based on change in CIMT. This can be avoided in the individual patient if determination of risk is based only on an observed change over time which is greater than the error of the method. To do this, providers need to use IMT vendors who have peer-reviewed data regarding the error of the method on their specific protocol, and their technicians.

The CAPTIVATE study is the last example of an individual study that showed benefit.

CAPTIVATE (Meuwese, 2009), the Carotid Atherosclerosis Progression Trial Investigating Vascular ACAT Inhibition Treatment Effects (CAPTIVATE), was a prospective, randomized, stratified, double-blind, placebo-controlled study looking at 892 patients heterozygous for familial hypercholesterolemia. The study was multicenter, conducted at 40 lipid clinics in the United States, Canada, Europe, South Africa, and Israel (Meuwese, 2009).

In this trial, participants received either 100 mg/d of pactimibe (n = 443) or matching placebo (n = 438), in addition to standard lipid-lowering therapy. The Maximum CIMT measurements did not show a pactimibe treatment effect (difference, 0.004 mm; 95% confidence interval [CI], −0.023 to 0.015 mm; P = .64); however, the less variable mean CIMT measurement revealed an increase of 0.014 mm (95% CI, −0.027 to 0.000 mm; P = .04) in patients administered pactimibe vs.

placebo. Major cardiovascular events (cardiovascular death, myocardial infarction, and stroke) also occurred more often in patients administered pactimibe vs. placebo (10/443 [2.3%] vs. 1/438 [0.2%]; P = .01).

The authors conclude: "In patients with familial hypercholesterolemia, pactimibe had no effect on atherosclerosis as assessed by changes in maximum CIMT compared with placebo but was associated with an increase in mean CIMT as well as increased incidence of major cardiovascular events." Once again, we see that the protocol matters.

In the MIDAS trial (Borhani, 1996), one of the studies included in the meta-analysis, isradipine compared with hydrochlorothiazide did not significantly slow the rate of progression of the intima-media thickening in the carotid arteries. In this study, blood pressure control was as follows: Systolic BP was slightly lower in the HCTZ group (19.5 mmHg lower than baseline, vs. 16 mm Hg for isradipine). Diastolic BP was lowered by 13 mmHg in both groups. About one half of the patients remained on the assigned monotherapy; about one quarter required the addition of enalapril.

There were 25 major clinical events in the isradipine leg and 14 in the HCTZ (p=0.07). The most common major event was angina pectoris (11 in the Isradipine vs. 3 in the HCTZ. There were no statistically significant differences in the number of major vascular procedures (11 vs 10), but there were 40 non-major vascular procedures in the Isradipine leg vs. 23 in the HCTZ group (p-0.02). Finally, there were 13 incidences of cancer in the Isradipine group vs. 20 in the HCTZ group (p=0.21). All-cause mortality was not statistically significant (8 vs. 9).

In an accompanying editorial, Aram Chobanian, MD (Boston University School of Medicine) noted that several design problems may have contributed to the failure of MIDAS to detect any effect of isradipine on the rate of progression of carotid atherosclerosis. The sample size was based on the rate of progression of IMT in a different population (patients with hypercholesterolemia, who were excluded in this trial); enalapril was added to a quarter of patients in both groups; systolic BP was better controlled in the HCTZ group; problems with ultrasound interpretation required a post-hoc correction.

As for the increase in vascular events, and angina in particular, Dr. Chobanian notes that a similar effect has been suggested in other studies which have looked at the use of calcium channel blockers for the treatment of coronary disease. Some evidence points to an adverse effect of short-acting dihydropyridines only, yet some point to an effect of all calcium channel blockers. Much of these data are case-control and thus inconclusive, and MIDAS was not designed to look at these issues specifically.

Nevertheless, the results do contribute to the evidence that caution should be exercised when prescribing calcium channel blockers, that the long-acting and non-dihydropyridines should be considered preferentially and that first-line therapy for hypertension should probably include other types of agents.

The take away as it relates to IMT is that one must be cautious in presuming a decrease in IMT can be construed to mean improved outcome if the agent being used for treatment is potentially harmful through some mechanism other than atherosclerosis. Nevertheless, this study is used in the meta-analysis to draw conclusions which are really not supported by the analysis.

To pool data from MIDAS (Borhani, 1996), which used max IMT from multiple segments and compared one antihypertensive to another, with data from CLAS (Azen, 1996) which took subjects who had already had a cardiovascular event and were being treated with two cholesterol lowering agents (niacin and colestipol) and looked only at far wall IMT cannot really be valid. It would be nearly impossible to draw any clear cut conclusion when comparing these two studies. Yet – these two meta-analysis did just that.

A meta-analysis that includes 41 studies each using different inclusion criteria, different protocols, different interventions and disparate technologies is disingenuous and intellectually dishonest. Though the biostatistical rigor was impressive, you simply can't realistically pool such disparate data and protocols and expect to get useful information.

In METEOR (Crouse, 2007) there were more clinical events in those treated with rosuvastatin than in those treated with placebo.

Yet, rosuvastatin slowed progression significantly more than placebo. Because the inclusion criteria required subjects to be at very low risk for events there were, indeed, few cardiovascular ischemic events (6 out of 987 subjects). This was not felt to be statistically significant. Yet, these events are included in the meta-analysis.

Taking the results of multiple intervention trials such as MIDAS (Borhani, 1996), ARBITER (Taylor, 2006), and METEOR (Crouse, 2007), none of which had enough clinical events within the individual study to correlate those events with change rate . . . each using disparate inclusion criteria, each using different treatment regimens and different protocols for scanning and reading, some of which used older technology (MIDAS 1996) and then pool that data with newer technology, and then trying to draw firm conclusions concerning the correlation of change rate with events is not just a complex task . . . it is not only ill-advised, but it is extremely doubtful that any conclusions would be valid or useful.

PLAQUE CHARACTERIZATION

The prognostic value of echolucent carotid plaques in stable CAD patients was studied. A group of 215 patients with stable CAD were followed from one to 30 months (mean 14) (Honda, 2004). Patients with echolucent (non-calcified) carotid plaques (n =112) had 29 coronary events during the follow-up period, whereas patients without echolucent plaques (n =103) had only four coronary events (p =0.001) (Table 3). All but one of the 29 coronary events in the total echolucent group (i.e., 97%) were recorded in patients diagnosed with stable CAD with multiple echolucent carotid plaques. There were no significant differences in the dosages of administered medications between the patients with and those without coronary events (data not shown). Kaplan-Meier analysis in patients with stable CAD demonstrated that the **presence of echolucent carotid plaques was associated with a significantly higher probability of developing coronary events** (p 0.001).

Not only was plaque ignored in many of the studies used by both of these meta-analysis, so was the echolucency, a sonographic finding which would appear to be of considerable clinical significance.

TAKE AWAY

Although the meta-analyses in AHJ and JACC cast doubt that serial monitoring is of value, very few of the studies in the meta-analysis were designed to answer this specific question; many lacked quality controls, and the majority were done with disparate protocols and using older technology. Plaque analysis was largely ignored. In contrast, many individual intervention studies have shown serial monitoring to be of benefit in assessing efficacy of treatment. Utilization of serial monitoring in an individual patient where data is acquired and analyzed in identical fashion year after year more closely approximates the individual studies showing benefit than the meta-analyses that did not.

Back to the question: Does serial monitoring of CIMT add to the predictive power of a single CIMT measurement?

In light of the importance of the presence of plaque, characterization of plaque as non-calcified or calcified (which is as nearly as accurate and reproducible as the measurements themselves), the constant improvement in technology and the readily achievable accuracy of 0.002mm in obtaining a scan in an office-based setting of an individual patient . . . the answer is clearly 'YES'.

These protocols may improve the ability not only of a baseline scan to predict risk, but allow the clinician to assess the progression of the atherosclerotic process. One must come to terms with the fact that an intervention may lead to a change in outcome independent of ultrasound changes if the treatment has an off-target beneficial or deleterious effect on the subject.

Finally, some studies specifically designed to assess its benefit clearly show the benefit of measuring change over time. Some of these studies are included in the meta-analysis, e.g., CLAS, Carotid Plaque Area. CAPTIVATE is not included in the meta-analysis but is reviewed above.

Since the atherosclerotic process is a focal abnormality, it is widely believed that circumferential scanning of all segments of the carotid artery provide a better estimate of the extent and severity of carotid atherosclerosis in an individual.

Several studies showed that Mean Maximum CIMT measurements can be obtained in practically all subjects in a reliable and reproducible manner. It has been proposed to use Mean Maximum CIMT as a primary CIMT outcome measurement in randomized clinical trials, with segment- specific CIMT measurements as secondary outcomes. Such an approach requires more time for image acquisition and reading phase compared with common carotid IMT measurements but is worth the additional effort.

It would appear that using the mean maximum CIMT (multiple segments) preferentially over mean common CIMT as the primary outcome in randomized clinical trials that are designed to evaluate the efficacy of pharmacological and nonpharmacological interventions is a scientifically sound recommendation. Guidelines for interpreting scan data and integrating it into a comprehensive treatment plan must be developed.

With agreement on standard scanning and reading protocols (what to measure, where to measure and how often to measure) that includes at least mean max measurements and average mean measurements in the common, followed by plaque interrogation in the internal, the bifurcation, the internal, external, and perhaps even the femoral arteries, B-mode ultrasound imaging of the arteries has the potential of becoming an indispensable tool to assess efficacy of treatment in the prevention of heart attack and stroke.

The protocol used by CardioRisk Laboratories and referred to in prospective, double-blind peer-reviewed literature is a more logical approach. CardioRisk's protocol includes Mean Max, and Avg Mean IMT measurements, and then a separate interrogation of the common carotid, the bifurcation of the common, the internal and external carotids to look for plaque as an independent process during the same patient scan. Femoral scans can be completed as well. Plaque that is imaged is then measured for volume and echogenicity for the degree of calcification. The combinations of measurement protocols in the common, the bifurcation of the common, the internal and external carotids and perhaps even the femoral arteries has the potential to increase the ability of B-mode ultrasound of the arteries to predict risk not only at baseline, but to monitor efficacy of therapy over time.

Certification of the process to assure accuracy at least to 0.002mm is conducted at regular intervals and all technicians must pass the double-blind, performance-based certification process. This process has been validated by the International Society of Clinical Intima-Media Ultrasonography (ISCIMU), the only organization to certify a medical test using double-blind performance-based certifications.

THE SCIENCE OF QUALITY MEASUREMENTS STANDARD DEVIATIONS, REPRODUCIBILITY, SENSITIVITY, AND SPECIFICITY AND WHY IT MATTERS!

There is a mathematical and, more to the point, a statistical term which many of us learned in school called the normal distribution sometimes referred to as the bell curve. Imbedded within that construct is another term I came to love and cherish as it defined much of the world I grew up in professionally. That term is Standard Deviation (SD).

There are certain phenomena that assume a normal distribution, such that the probability of an event occurring within a range of values is estimated to be equivalent to the area under the curve represented by the range of values. Conceptually you will remember that many or even most things that can be physically measured fall under this normal distribution often referred to as just "the area under the curve". Explicit in this construct is the fact that approximately 68% of estimated values that can be physically measured fall within plus or minus one standard deviation. Approximately 95% of the estimated values of anything that can be physically measured fall within plus or minus two standard deviations, and just over 99% of the estimated values of anything that can be physically measured will fall into the area under the curve plus or minus 3 standard deviations (Figure 1).

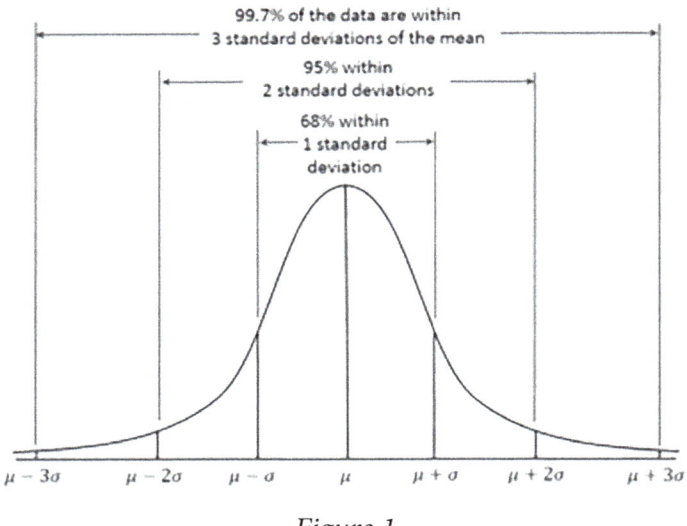

Figure 1

Standard deviation is a mathematical equation used to measure the distance from the mean of any group of measurements or data points. It is arrived at by taking the square root of the squared difference from the mean, divided by the number of observations minus one (Figure 2).

$$S_x = \sqrt{\frac{\sum_{i=1}^{n}(x_i - \bar{x})^2}{n-1}}$$

n = The number of data points

$\bar{x}$ = The mean of the x_i

x_i = Each of the values of the data

Figure 2

The relevance of that information cannot be overstated. We use that construct in virtually every scientific article or publication that has been in print since the beginning of the 20th century. It is the science that determines statistical validity and statistical significance.

Standard deviation helps us to better understand variation in data, and the significance or reproducibility of the data from any sample size. The 95% confidence interval we have come to cherish as the minimum threshold for statistical significance is predicated on this science. The confidence interval is a function, or a calculation derived from the deviation from the population mean of the sample being measured.

The reported margin of error of a survey or poll is calculated from the standard error of the mean – which is a function (the inverse of the square root of the sample size) or in other words, it is the product of the standard deviation. Another way to think about the Standard Error of the Mean (SEM) is that the formula for SEM is the standard deviation divided by the square root of the sample size. This requires us to first square the difference between each data point and the sample mean and find the sum of those values. This tells us the amount of deviation. Then, we divide that sum by the sample size minus one to show the variance. Finally, we take the square root of the variance to get the Standard Deviation. The SEM and SD are different, but essential elements to understanding the data in every sample we measure. We literally use this math and the construct of standard deviation in virtually every piece of publishable science.

The good news is you don't need to know these formulas to use them effectively. There are plenty of software products, including those in the public domain that will automatically do the math and calculate the standard deviation for you. That said, we should understand some basic effects of the standard deviation.

Another way to think of or visualize the effect of standard deviation is to imagine that the more variation there is, the wider the distribution curve, the more attenuated the slope of the curve, the higher the SD. Standard deviation is expressed in the same units as the data being measured, which makes it particularly useful (Figure 3). The figure below is labeled "Gaussian Distribution", named after Carl Friedrich Gauss who used it in 1809 for the analysis of astronomical data on positions. It is important to note that Gaussian Distribution is synonymous to Normal Distribution, and bell curve. An interesting side note is that Abraham de Moivre, the French-born mathematician, was the first to describe the normal distribution as an approximation to the binomial, and a pioneer in the development of analytic geometry and the theory of probability. Also in the diagram below, and for your reference, the symbol σ signifies standard deviation and the symbol μ or mu is the symbol for the exact center of the normal distribution or the mean.

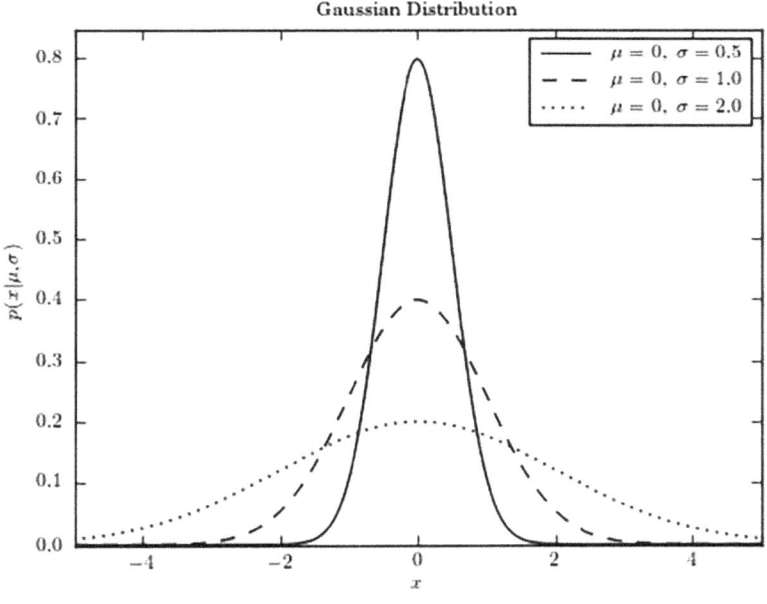

Figure 3

On a personal note, while attempting to pay my way through graduate school, I did a lot of consulting with manufacturers using standard deviation to evaluate and fix manufacturing issues. Standard deviation has the unique ability to measure the variability of a process in real time. We used standard deviation to quickly identify manufacturing issues in real time.

Let's say, for example, that the widgets being manufactured are Coke can lids (the top of the can which is subsequently fastened to the top and the bottom of a Coke can). Measuring the size of the hole through which this delicious elixir would be sipped has to conform to certain size parameters. This should be self-evident. The parameters are very tiny. If the size of the hole is too big or too small by more than an extremely tight threshold, then the lid fails to seal and the soda will leak out the top of the can. If you are a Coke distributor or bottler, that is NOT a good thing. As a result, when a process is reliable, the standard deviation of the measured outcomes of the process will be small. If there is a high degree of variability, the process will be considered unreliable and the standard deviation will be larger.

By measuring in real time several key characteristics of our lid we can quickly identify any finished goods that are one or two standard deviations away from the mean. In other words, if there is too much variation in the finished product from the original design . . . and from the mean of the other widgets being produced, then that widget would fail our quality system. Of course, care needs to be made to make sure that measurements are taken the same way, at the same location, every time, or the method will fail. More to that point later.

This technique is utilized by manufacturers of a wide variety of products, and truthfully, by any manufacturer who cares about the quality of the thing they are going to produce. When a product or widget falls out of these tight parameters, they should be pulled off the manufacturing line.

From a quality standpoint, the goal is to sharpen the slope of the distribution curve so that there is very little difference between the mean (the center line of the distribution curve) and the outer two lines. The steeper the curve or the slope of the curve, the higher the quality and the less variation there is in whatever is being manufactured. So, in the case of our Coke can lid, a steeper sloped curve means that there is very little variation between the lids. The sharper and steeper the slope of the bell-shaped curve, the less variation in the manufacturing process, which translates to a better or higher quality of the widget being produced.

That was the beauty of it . . . it didn't really matter what the widget was that was being manufactured. So long as you were measuring the correct aspects of whatever widget you were producing, and so long as you were consistent in how and where you measured those widgets, the principles of standard deviation would make it better!

This type of process for quality control and quality assurance is known as Statistical Process Control (SPC). Statistical Process Control is a method of quality control which employs statistical method to monitor and control the process. It is the process of making things better via the scientific construct of standard deviation and normative distribution (e.g. statistical method).

What I came to love about this science is that it applied to virtually anything and everything that is made. You can use these principles of statistical process control and standard deviation to improve the quality of anything that is manufactured and virtually any product, service, or process.

In medicine we use it to track outcomes. Standard deviation is used to track efficacy of medications or technologies. We use the science of statistical variation in virtually every aspect of patient interaction. This science is the basis for actuary tables and insurance rates. It is a big, beautiful, and infinitely useful science.

GAMES PLAYED WITH STATISTICS

In the case of CIMT – this science has never been more important or relevant. However, . . . it is not the ONLY science we need to be concerned with.

Smart people figured out a long time ago that if all we care about is reproducibility, or in minimizing variability, then we can easily design a protocol which addresses the issue. Since standard deviation is a function of the sample size and normative distribution, we can minimize the effects of variation owing to the disparity in the quality of the images taken between different operators and readers, by increasing the sample size.

The way to minimize the effects of variation is to simply take more measurements. Taking more measurements minimizes the effects on variability owing to sonographers and readers of different skill levels.

Unfortunately, when you take too many measurements, you can also minimize the effects of variation owing to pathology. This can have an unintended and dangerous consequence by taking the plaque right out of the equation so that the effect of a large plaque on the mean of a sample is nearly irrelevant – a rounding error.

Indeed – significantly increasing the number of measurements will almost always reduce the degree of variability. Unfortunately, this approach has a potentially fatal flaw in that the more measurements we take, the more we increase the risk of minimizing the effects of abnormal findings (i.e. a large plaque) on the total sample. It is a delicate balance that must be struck between reproducibility, and sensitivity (e.g. the ability to see abnormal results from pathology within the average mean of a sample of multiple angles, when the pathology only appears in a single frame or image).

We have seen some CIMT vendors who not only take so many images and measurements that they completely nueter the ability to correctly identify pathology, but then they then assign 3 or more readers to read the same images from which they once again take an average mean and report them as a finding. Although this method would be very reproducible, it is nearly completely invalid as a tool to correctly identify disease. An average of an average of an average is invalid as a diagnostic tool.

In the case of a technology such as Carotid Intima Media Thickness (CIMT) where the walls we are measuring are expressed in hundredths of millimeters, and the variability between measurements can be in the thousandths of millimeters, the reproducibility matters, but so does sensitivity.

In the landmark Atherosclerosis Results in Community Study (The ARIC study), the average thickness of a normal and healthy artery was 0.60mm (Chambless, 1997).   Let's use this measurement to illustrate how reproducibility, and sensitivity interact.

THE EFFECT OF MEASUREMENTS ON CIMT PROTOCOL AND RESULTS

In our example lets imagine that the average mean of a series of measurements (n) of the intima-media layers in a person's common carotid artery measure exactly the same at 0.61mm. All but 10 of these measurements are the same at 0.61mm.

Obviously, this could never happen, but it is an important intellectual exercise to better understand the effects of sample size. The 10 measurement exceptions, which did not measure 0.61mm, but measured 3.5mm each, represent an area where plaque was found. So, in the area of the plaque lesion, 10 X measurements were taken, each measuring exactly 3.5mm.

Let's further assume that this average mean is derived from n measurements, from 3 different companies where n = 100, 1,000, or 10,000 measurements respectively. These measurements were taken from a single patient, at multiple angles, on both the patient's right and left carotid arteries.

So, let's also assume for the sake of ease in calculation that we can take a maximum of 100 measurements per image and that these measurements cover an area approximating a 1cm segment of the patient's artery. So, if we wanted to increase the number of measurements, we need only increase the number of images.

Suppose now that we want to look at both the left and the right carotid arteries because we are interested in creating a more complete picture of the amount of systemic inflammation found in the arterial wall. We are essentially looking for a composite picture as to the state of each patient's arterial health.

Now imagine that we are evaluating several scan protocols by several different well-meaning imaging companies. Company #1 will take 50 measurements from the images of the left artery, and 50 measurements from the right for a total of 100 measurements. To keep it simple, we separately take 10 measurements of a plaque, each measuring 3.5mm (that is a large plaque!). Company #2 will take a total of 1000 measurements plus the 10 plaque measurements, and Company #3 will take a total of 10,000 measurements plus the 10 plaque measurements. Let us now take a look at the effect on reproducibility and sensitivity as represented by each of these three protocols. (Table 1)

Table 1

	Company #1	Company #2	Company #3
Number of Measurements	100	1000	10000
Area of Plaque = 3.5 X 10	35	35	35
Sum of normal measurement	100 X 0.61 61	1000 X 0.61 610	10,000 X 0.61 6100
Sum of Plaque measurements	10 X 3.5 35	10 X 3.5 35	10 X 3.5 35
Sum of All Measurements	96	645	6135
Average Mean of All measurements	0.96	0.645	0.6135

What should be immediately apparent is that those companies that used too many measurements are unable to differentiate the arteries of someone who has significant inflammation from those who do not (see highlighted cells at the bottom of Table 1).

In the example above, the 10 X 3.5mm measurements of plaque barely amount to a rounding error when compared to the other measurements (of 0.61mm) from *Company #3*'s protocol. *Company #3* reports the Average of the Mean as 0.6135mm – an insignificant and negligible change from a healthy artery (0.61mm). *Company #2* does a better job, but if our standard deviation is > 0.015, they also will be unable to determine whether or not the artery has increased or decreased the amount of inflammation, much less demonstrate an abnormality indicative of the large atherosclerotic plaque in this patient's artery. At least not at the 95% confidence level. [(0.645 ± (0.015 X 2)]) - where 0.015mm is the standard deviation and 2 X the SD is used to arrive at a 95% confidence interval. Only the measurement from *Company* 1 shows the significant abnormality. They report an average mean of 0.96mm and correctly identify this segment as significantly above the normal range.

Even though this example grossly oversimplifies the issues surrounding reproducibility and sensitivity, it does underscore the need for a scientific approach to protocol design. It gets MUCH more complicated. We haven't even begun the discussion of skew, kurtosis, or goodness of fit.

We should also assume that it is nearly impossible physiologically to get an ultrasonic measurement from the exact same place in three-dimensional space. Many have tried using protractor-like gauges to provide guidance of the ultrasonic transducer, but even this fails to do much except provide a slight improvement in getting the transducer to a routine location on the outside of a patient's neck.

Unfortunately, human anatomy varies quite a bit. Some patient's internal carotids present themselves in a superior position to the external artery, and others present themselves inferior to the external vessel. The arteries themselves often present themselves at different depths. Some vessels are tortuous and look like a snake as they weave inside the patient's neck. All these issues create variability which, absent a specific scientifically derived imaging protocol, can affect the reproducibility of the images in the scan.

Since this is the reality so far as our current understanding, we must assume that measurements from different angles will result in disparate measurements in our results, especially if only single or minimal number of measurements are taken. Too many measurements will likely diminish or completely annul the tests' ability to register the effect of atherosclerotic plaque in the average of the mean. This has the net effect of minimizing the procedure's ability to correctly identify patients at increased risk for future events. All of these have been addressed in the vast array of literature – which have led some in the scientific community to distance themselves from the testing modality entirely. This is sad, because these issues can all be addressed scientifically.

If we question this, we need look no further than an article published in Atherosclerosis back in 2013 which influenced the United States Preventative Services Task Force (USPSTF) to not recommend CIMT for routine use. The USPSTF soured on CIMT technology based on a large meta-analysis which tried to make some sort of sense of 30 different IMT studies, each utilizing a different protocol. While the statistical efforts were laudable in terms of biostatistical prowess, the study ignored the first rule of science: "Garbage in = Garbage out". No amount of biostatistical magic can fix that problem. You simply can't compare the results from even two studies whose underlying protocols vary in the crucial methodologies and which affect their validity and reproducibility, much less 30.

Here is the point I hope you will take away from this chapter: absent a clearly defined written protocol which is scientifically designed and religiously adhered to, CIMT is powerless to inform a provider about disease status in any meaningful way. Power statistics should be used to identify the ideal sample size (number of measurements) to balance the importance of reproducibility with that of sensitivity. Absent a closely prescribed protocol which is religiously adhered to, the probability of false positive, or conversely, false negative results is significantly increased. When it comes to patient treatment recommendations, neither of these conditions is an acceptable alternative.

Unfortunately, many companies and individual sonographers who offer CIMT, simply do not know what they do not know. All you need to do is to make sure that the company you use has clearly defined protocols for both acquiring images and for reading or measuring them.

Here is the good news, you don't need to worry about any of that. The protocol used by CardioRisk Laboratories, and developed by Dr. Gene Bond is a protocol designed by science. Gene Bond was the author of the CIMT protocol used by the ARIC and other landmark CIMT epidemiologic studies. In a peer reviewed, prospective, double blind trial which involved different sonographers, different readers, and different equipment, the published reproducibility by CardioRisk Laboratories on an arithmetic basis was 0.002mm (Riches, 2010). The standard deviation was 0.02mm.

This protocol was useful and reproducible to successfully identify atherosclerotic plaque and to then characterize that plaque echogenically as being soft and echoluscent (e.g. vulnerable to rupture), heterogenous (less vulnerable, but still unstable), or hard and completely echogenic. At least one of these independent variables was significant in virtually every one of the large-scale studies involving CIMT.

TAKE AWAY:

If you want to use CIMT in your practice, you want it to be valid, reproducible, and preferably performed by technicians whose proficiency has been demonstrated in a double blind, performance-based certification. Every single CardioRisk Laboratories technician successfully passed a double-blind certification which was validated by the International Society of Clinical Intima Media Ultrasonography (ISCIMU).

Implementation

So, you've decided to implement advanced blood, functional, and/or structural testing in your office. The thought may have occurred to you: "what do I do now". Fortunately, that is the easy part. To begin with, you can download our free Implementation worksheet by navigating to the webpage: www.cardiorisk.us/gettingstarted.

Here you will find a very simple 4-step process which I have outlined for you below. What I want you to understand is that whether you are implementing all these tests, or any one of the tests . . . the process is extremely easy.

STEP 1: SIGNED AGREEMENTS

In order to get started with any vendor, you should probably have a written agreement. This protects you, and it protects your vendor. Vendor's that don't provide a written agreement should be avoided because they put you and your medical license at risk.

If you work with CardioRisk Laboratories, their simple two-page agreement spells out clearly what you are responsible for and what they are responsible for. Beyond that, it simply states that you will pay your bill in a timely way. It should probably be stated that you won't pay anything for these tests or services until you have been paid. The invoice from CardioRisk comes with your Patient Results and is not due for 30 days. In most cases this leaves more than enough time for you to collect payment from your patients or even 3rd party payers.

Generally, you will simply agree to aggregate a group of patients one day each week, each month, or each quarter . . . or on some other schedule which suits you and your practice. This is completely optional and up to you and your practice.

To make the business model work for all involved, you want to try to aggregate at least 20 patients for each visit by your vendor. This is less than ½ day of scanning time, and it can take place on a day you are not even in the office. Experience has shown that if you are presenting the opportunity for these tests using the scripts provided, even a concierge practice of only 200 patients will not have any trouble putting together multiple days of scanning each year.

In addition to their standard agreement, you should insist your vendor's sign and comply with a Business Associate Agreement which is a HIPAA requirement. If you plan on sharing patient data, you will want to have all vendors sign such an agreement. Absent this agreement, you and they will be in violation of the HIPPA laws should you share any patient data. This could be an extremely expensive mistake, which could put your practice at jeopardy. Once again, CardioRisk Laboratories provides this agreement as part of their standard operating procedures.

STEP 2: SCHEDULE TESTING DATES

It will be nearly impossible to line up patients or to get them excited about any test if you can't provide them with the specific date(s) and times that are available for the exam. You wouldn't expect them to sign up for a wellness exam absent this information, and it is naïve to expect them to sign up for any testing procedure absent this information.

Because of this, the next step is to pencil some dates on the calendar that work for your office. Ideally, these dates should coincide with a time and date when you have an extra room or rooms so that the testing does not interfere with your daily operations. Most of the accounts at CardioRisk Laboratories schedule an entire year of exam dates. This allows them to redirect patients who are not available for one scan date, to another or the next available scan date and time. This practice is crucial if you want the operation to run smoothly and you are to make this a normal part of your practice's offerings.

Many offices find that posting these dates for people to see enhances the visibility of the tests, and can provide a subtle reminder to patients about the availability of these tests. It is quite common for offices to post the availability of Flu or Shingles vaccines, for example. Letting people know of the availability of scan dates, encourages them to ask questions about whether or not they should consider having the exam.

STEP 3: TRAIN YOUR STAFF

One of the most overlooked steps in many medical practices is the need to thoroughly train staff. This is especially true when implementing a new test or protocol. The training does not need to take weeks or months, but staff should be made aware of at least the following:

- What are these tests?
- Why is the doctor recommending I get them?
- Why are these tests important?
- Who should get the test?
- Possible results or outcomes (so they can direct patients to next steps).
- Are the tests covered by Medicare and 3rd party payers – and if so, under what circumstances
- Scripts – what do you want your staff to say about the test when asked? (They will be asked)

Given that these questions will be asked, I have outlined this information below so that you can conduct your own Inservice . . . or you can use it as follow-up material pursuant to an Inservice by the staff at CardioRisk. This information is meant to be shared with your staff and can even be used as mini scripts they can utilize when responding to patient questions. In our experience with offices, most of the questions will relate to the functional and structural testing. Accordingly, these are the tests which are addressed below.

WHAT ARE THESE TESTS?

Endothelial Function – The EndoTherm Endothelial Function test is a physiologic test which measures your vascular function. You've probably had a blood pressure test – which is another kind of physiological test – the EndoTherm test provides unique insight in that we compare your right arm to your left arm. The test is performed while laying down and takes less than 30 minutes to perform. It can be completed at the same time as the CIMT exam. Blood pressure cuffs are placed on your arm. The cuff on your right arm is inflated for a 5-minute period. Upon release, we measure the amount of blood flow in the cuffed arm and compare it to the arm that was uncuffed. This provides unique insight into how well your circulatory responds to stress – a direct measure of vascular function. Vascular function provides the earliest warning of cardio and cerebrovascular disease – the disease responsible for most heart attacks and strokes. Vascular function is also the first to respond to therapy (e.g. medication and/or lifestyle changes). Like many blood tests, the patient should be fasting for at least 4 hours before taking the test. Patients may take most of their medications as directed . . . they should be in a 'steady state' at the time of the test. The exception to this would be any vasodilative drugs such as Viagra or Cialis – these types of medications should be avoided for at least 12 hours or at least one half life before the test.

CIMT (Structural Test) – The Carotid Intima Media Thickness test is an ultrasound test which measures the amount of disease found in the walls of your artery. It is a painless ultrasound exam, there are no needle sticks, no disrobing is required, and no radiation exposure from the exam. The test takes less than 15 minutes of your time and can be completed at the same time as the Endothelial Function exam. The test is performed while the patient is laying down. A small amount of water-soluble ultrasound gel is placed on the neck to conduct the sound waves. This gel will be removed at the end of the exam. Several hundred measurements are taken of the images collected at the time of the exam and results are mailed back to the office in about 5 business days. We call this 'the pregnancy test of heart disease' because of its accuracy. In a 10-year, 100,000-person-year study it caught 98.6% of the heart attacks and strokes before they happened. We simply don't have another test that is more accurate than this.

WHY IS THE DOCTOR RECOMMENDING THESE TESTS?

Heart attacks and Strokes are the #1 leading cause of death. They are currently responsible for more deaths than the next 3 leading causes of death combined . . . including all deaths from any form of cancer, and all deaths from any type of accident. Since most of these events are preventable, our office is committed to preventing these events from occurring in our patient population. These two tests provide additional information and insight not provided by the tests required by the current standard of care. We believe they provide unique insight to your current and future risk of events, while providing safe guidance on the efficacy of any treatment or intervention.

WHY ARE THESE TESTS IMPORTANT?

The tests required in the current standard of care miss a large percentage of the patients who go on to have a heart attack and/or stroke. We are committed to preventing these events in our patient population. These tests provide unique insight not provided by any other test in our office. They are an important part of the optimal care we strive to provide our patients. You do want optimal care, don't you?

WHO SHOULD GET THE TEST?

We recommend that all adult patients over the age of 30 get these tests at least once. If you are from southeast Asia, India, or you come from African/American decent . . . you should consider getting the test even earlier because patients from these genetic backgrounds tend to get the disease more often, and at an earlier age. The tests are repeated every 3 to 5 years in patients with normal results, and annually in patients with abnormal findings.

POSSIBLE RESULTS OR OUTCOMES (SO THEY CAN DIRECT PATIENTS TO NEXT STEPS).

Both of these tests report patient results in a Red, Yellow, and Green light panel or panels where Green is normal, and Yellow or Red are abnormal. A more thorough explanation of results and their meaning is provided in a subsequent chapter.

ARE THE TESTS COVERED BY MEDICARE AND 3RD PARTY PAYERS – AND IF SO, UNDER WHAT CIRCUMSTANCES

Both of these tests are covered in patients with known disease, and especially in those patients who have already exhibited signs and symptoms. We strongly encourage these patients to use these tests annually to enable us to continue to monitor their disease. Unfortunately, the test is rarely paid for as a screening tool where it has the capacity to save lives. Over half of those who have a heart attack or stroke had no signs or symptoms until they had their event. For this reason, we believe these tests are important for ALL adult patients. Medicare and other 3rd party payers rarely pay for optimal care. You do want optimal care, don't you?

SCRIPTS THAT WORK

Front Office to Patient (when presented with a prescription for the tests):

> "Oh good, these are two of the easiest tests you'll ever have. Our next testing day is on _____, we have time available at _____ or at _____ would either of those times work for you? Great, we look forward to seeing you then. Make sure to wear loose fitting clothing so that we can easily take your blood pressure and put an ultrasound wand on your neck."

Staff should be familiar with all the information presented above so that they can communicate it as needed when responding to questions from patients. CardioRisk can provide all of the information above in short two-page 'cheat sheets' which can be provided at no charge upon request.

STEP 4: BEGIN RECOMMENDING THESE TESTS TO YOUR PATIENTS

So, of all of the steps which are most important – this step trumps them all. If the provider does not recommend the test, it will never be utilized. We understand that often patients come to a medical office in search of answers to unrelated questions. We understand that your time with each patient is extremely limited and that you have a list of objectives which must be accomplished during each patient engagement or interaction. Having said that, if you don't find a way to introduce a short script about cardiovascular wellness, your patients will never get these life-saving procedures. We must find ways to direct each patient's optimal care . . . even if/when it interrupts the dialogue they so often want to have with you. With this in mind, we have prepared several easy, short, and simple to implement scripts you can add to any patient interaction. We have empirical data to show these scripts work. We are confident if you use them, you will find many people signing up for the new tests and you will be offering better care to your patients.

RECOMMENDED PATIENT SCRIPTS: (WWW.CARDIORISK.US/PATIENTSCRIPTS)

Provider to Patient:

"We ought to check your risk for heart attack and/or stroke – I'd like you to have a CIMT and an endothelial function exam. These are two of the easiest tests you'll ever have. Please tell the front desk to schedule you for your CIMT . . . (hand them a script for the tests)"

Now . . . if the patient looks to you for additional information, please add this to your script:

> "The CIMT test is a non-invasive ultrasound test that checks your risk for heart attack and stroke. In a 10- year, 100,000 person-year study, the IMT test caught 98.6% of the heart attacks and strokes before they happened. Quite frankly, I don't have another test in my toolbox that is more effective at finding those patients at risk . . . and in most cases, it finds them in time to treat them medically, so they don't need to be treated surgically."

> "The Endothelial Function test measures any physiological loss of vascular function. It provides me with the earliest assessment of cardiovascular risk."

> "Just take this script to the front desk and they can help you get these tests scheduled."

Take-Aways

That's it – A four step process to easily integrate these tests into your practice. A vendor should be willing to hold your hand through each of these steps – but one thing is sure . . . the longer you wait to take the first step . . . the longer your patients will wait for these life-saving procedures.

Albert Einstein once defined insanity as "Doing the same thing over and over again and expecting a different result". You have now seen the data in favor of the use of these tests. You are also aware of the fundamental weaknesses in the current standard of care as it relates to this disease. It is compelling. Your patients are counting on you to provide them with Optimal Care. If not now . . . when? When will your work life be any less stressful? When will you have more time than right now.

The choice is always yours – but I urge you to wait no longer. Pick up the phone and make the call. To make it stupid simple . . . let me help you.

Just text the letters **"CIMT"** to this number: **650-525-2250**

That's it – that will launch a series of contacts with you. Within minutes of sending that text, you will receive a contact from my office asking you to follow a link which will only ask you a few questions about your practice: The Business Name, the Office Address, Your Name, and a contact phone number.

Once we have that information you will receive a follow-up text from my staff confirming we received your information. Very shortly your office will receive a call from someone at CardioRisk providing your staff with all the information you will need to get started. You may want to give them a heads up that this call will be coming.

I don't know how to make it any easier for you. Take the next step. Send us the text. You are where you are because you get things done. You are a person who takes action. Here is the information again:

To Bring CIMT Into Your Practice

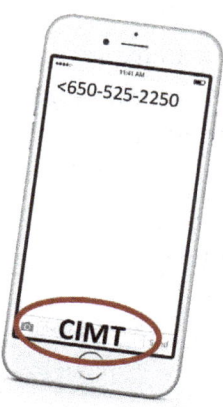

TEXT:
"CIMT"
650-525-2250

This will help us to follow up with you and to help you schedule an appointment

Interpretation of Results

I spend a fair amount of my time speaking to physicians about the test results from various vendors. Indeed, not all CIMT results are created equal, and many of the reports can be confusing to the uninitiated. Over the years I have found it easier to start explanations from the "20,000-foot level" to make sure everyone begins with the same foundation. In the pages that follow, I have tried to capture the essence of that information so that you can refer to these pages whenever you are looking at CIMT results. It should be stated up front that while I am an expert on the reports generated from CardioRisk, I do not pretend to be an expert on reports provided by other vendors. I hope this information may still be useful in helping you better understand results no matter who is providing them.

We have already discussed disease progression in a previous chapter. However, to better understand the results, we should review a few basic tenets of the disease in order to better understand data in these reports which could be confusing.

For all intents and purposes, this disease begins in the blood. We could argue that it begins with lifestyle choices, etc., but the first empirical evidence we see will be in bio monitors (e.g. pathogens in the blood). When a concentration of a particular pathogen like cholesterol aggregates in a deciliter of blood, the probability of those pathogens penetrating the structural wall of the artery increases. Left alone, these pathogens will eventually penetrate and perforate the endothelial lining of the arterial wall. When conditions are right, these pathogens get trapped inside the intima of the arterial wall. The subsequent sequelae associated with the penetration and trapping of a pathogen into the wall of the artery is phagocytosis. In this process, monocytes traveling in the white cells of the blood also penetrate the endothelial lining. When they find a pathogen that shouldn't be there, they penetrate the endothelium and activate themselves into macrophages. The macrophages begin to consume these pathogens. Macrophages consume until they literally explode. The by-product of this cascade of events are foam cells and fatty streaks within the arterial wall . . . inflammation. Since our arteries are part of the sympathetic nervous system, we can't feel this inflammation of the arterial wall. The inflammation can cause bulging of the inner wall towards the lumen, but just as often, perhaps even more often, the bulging occurs away from the lumen. In either case, the result of this process is a weakening of the arterial wall. Eventually, if left untreated, this inflammation will aggregate into a white puss-like material, very similar to an acne lesion – only on the 'skin' of the arterial wall. Much like facial acne, when they first form, they are soft, whitehead-like lesions which are extremely vulnerable to rupture. Over time, if they don't rupture, calcium and other minerals will attract to the surface of the lesion providing additional stability. A healed plaque becomes completely encased in a thick and tough calcific shell which is highly unlikely to rupture. Armed with this understanding – we are better prepared to interpret the results from the CardioRisk Patient Results Report. Below is a 5-step process to interpret these results.

See **Table 2.** It is important to note that a high-risk patient in a Primary or Secondary prevention environment is not the same as a high-risk patient at the cardiologist or neurologist's office. For starters, none of these finding (with one exception prominently annotated below) are candidates for a surgical intervention requiring the intervention of a cardiologist or other surgeon. These patients will be treated using medical vs. surgical interventions (lifestyle and pharmacological).

Table 2

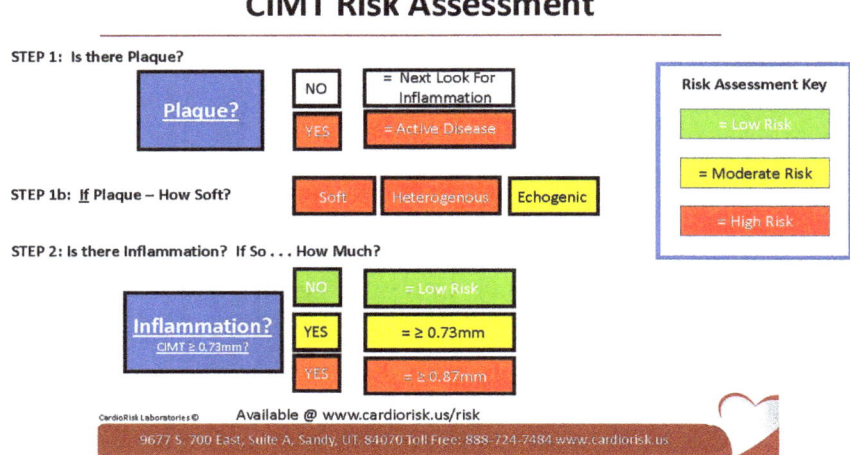

For context, we always begin the CIMT risk assessment by looking at the most important risk factors and then working progressively downward to the less relevant risk factors.

1) Plaque/No Plaque: The most important finding on any report is the plaque/no plaque question. This data is found on the report under the heading "Plaque Burden", and it has two conditions: Red or Green (e.g. Plaque, no Plaque). Patients with plaque have the same approximate risk as someone who has already experienced a heart attack or stroke (Bots, 1997). Given this information, a patient where plaque is found as a function of their ultrasound exam, should be treated as a high-risk patient – in the same way you would treat any patient who had already experienced a heart attack or stroke. This value is expressed as plaque burden and has only two conditions: Red (the patient has plaque) or Green (no plaque was found). **Table 3**

Table 3

| Date of Birth: | 11/11/1943 |
| Referring Physician: | DR. SAMPLE |

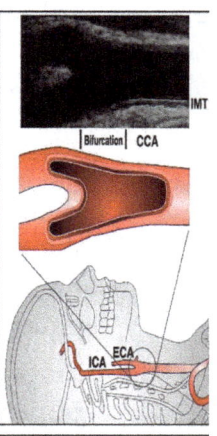

Patient Age	74	Patient IMT	0.73 mm
Arterial Age	58	Normal IMT	< .50 mm

		CV Event Risk			All measurements in mm	
Test Criteria:	Normal	Moderate	High	Last Visit (2015)†	Alert Value*
Early Event Risk⁺⁺	2.0				3
Average CCA Mean IMT		0.73			0.73
Average CCA Max Region		0.81			0.75
Plaque Burden**			2.0		

Comments: The following values are the largest intima-media thickness (IMT) measurements found in each carotid artery segment. Any measurement equal to or 1.3mm is defined as 'plaque' and is characterized as being: S = Soft; H = Heterogeneous; or E = Echogenic (includes mineral deposits like calcium). All measurements are in millimeters.

Right CCA .8; Bulb .7; Internal Carotid .7
Left CCA .8 Bulb 2.0 E; nternal Carotid .7
Doppler was used bilaterally.

2) Echogenicity of Plaque: The next question is to determine the relative echogenicity. To address this question, our eyes should drop to the Comments section of the results. In the comments section you will find the single largest IMT measurement in each of the 6 – 8 segments measured.

Every CardioRisk exam interrogates the common carotid, the bifurcation of the common carotid, and the internal carotid artery. Some offices ask us to also interrogate the external carotid and/or the femoral arteries on new patients, in order to assess plaque development in as many vascular beds as is prudent. In both the Cafes-Cave study, and our own internal research, adding femoral artery IMT interrogation to the exam catches an additional 10 – 18% of the infected but asymptomatic population. It is a prudent step, particularly in new patients where no plaque can be found in their carotid arteries, but where there is some evidence of inflammation. Femoral Intima-Media Thickness scanning is unnecessary in patients where plaque was clearly identified in the carotids. In the comments section of the report, all IMT measurements ≥ 1.3mm will have a letter next to it. These letters designate the plaque as

S = Soft. These plaques are the most dangerous because they are prone to rupture;

H = Heterogenous. These plaques have begun the healing process and have begun to show calcific changes demonstrated by white speckle in the core of the lesion. They are not, however, completely healed and they are still at increased risk of future rupture;

E = Echogenic. These plaques are completely healed. The amount of mineral buildup around the lesion is so dense that they cast an ultrasonic shadow (the sound waves can't even penetrate). These plaques are much more stable and highly unlikely to rupture. At the very least there is little more that can be done for them clinically. In our experience (> 150MM IMT measurements at the time of this book's printing) these plaques will not disappear via anything but a surgical removal. From a clinical standpoint, we recommend continued monitoring and management of any conditions that led to plaque formation in the first place.

3) Inflammation: The next factor affecting risk is the amount of inflammation found in the arterial wall. This data is found in two boxes: Average CCA Mean IMT and Average CCA Max Region. The difference between these two metrics is not tangential. The Average CCA Mean is the average mean of approximately 600 measurements from 6 different angles (3 distinct angles on the Right carotid and 3 distinct angles on the Left carotid) in the distal one centimeter of the common carotid artery.

As atherosclerosis is a rough disease, and atherosclerotic inflammation is almost always characterized by very small rises and falls in the arterial wall, the Average CCA Mean IMT captures both the peaks and the valleys. The Average CCA Max Region measurement, by contrast, captures the 6 highest 0.10mm peaks (one 0.10mm peak from each of 6 distinct angles). A recent publication of our data conducted by Dr.'s Amy Doneen and Bradley Bale in conjunction with Johns Hopkins University (Cheng, 2016) found that the delta between these two measurements is important. Management of the delta between these two measurements towards homogeneity is an important marker of treatment success. Table 4 The larger the delta between these two values, the greater the risk of atherosclerotic disease and subsequent clinical events.

Table 4

Date of Birth: /1947
Referring Physician:

Patient Age	70	Patient IMT	1.35 mm
Arterial Age	>80	Normal IMT	< 50 mm

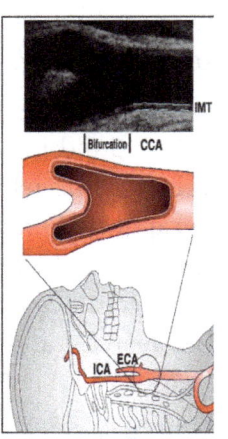

IMT

Bifurcation | CCA

ECA
ICA

Test Criteria:	CV Event Risk			Last Visit (2016)†	Alert Value*
	Normal	Moderate	High		All measurements in mm
Early Event Risk⁺⁺			3.6		2.5
Average CCA Mean IMT			1.35		0.73
Average CCA Max Region			1.65		0.75
Plaque Burden**			14.1		

Comments: The following values are the largest intima-media thickness (IMT) measurements found in each carotid artery segment. Any measurement equal to or 1.3mm is defined as 'plaque' and is characterized as being: S = Soft; H = Heterogeneous; or E = Echogenic (includes mineral deposits like calcium). All measurements are in millimeters.

Right CCA 2.3 H; Bulb 3.2 E; Internal Carotid 3.6 E
Left CCA 1.1; Bulb 2.6 E; Internal Carotid 2.4 E
Doppler was used bilaterally.

4) Arterial Age. This number can be found at the top of the report, just underneath the patient's chronological age. No alert value is associated with this metric because it is a relative risk score. This value is a coefficient of the Average CCA Mean IMT measurement. It is useful to help patients understand what the absolute values found in both the Average CCA Mean IMT and the Average CCA Max Region means to them at a personal level. Since some of the patients you will be screening will be younger, and will have no increased risk based on their absolute risk factors (e.g. Plaque Burden; Average CCA Mean IMT, and Average CCA Max Region), this value is there to help patients navigate the relationship of those other values in relation to their own situation. They may be progressing faster or slower than other patients in longitudinal and epidemiological studies. It is useful to understand whether each patient is progressing faster or slower than the patients in clinical studies. However, this value should not be used by clinicians to monitor disease as no data exists connecting Arterial Age to increase risk of future events. The raw measurements found in both the Average CCA Mean IMT and the Average CCA Max Region both have alert values next to them because these alert values do correlate to increased risk as presented in multiple epidemiologic and longitudinal studies.

5) Early Event Risk. This value is derived from the thickest IMT value found in any of the images taken from multiple angles on either the right or left carotid arteries. Its implication is one of the more complicated metrics on the CardioRisk Scan Patient Results report. The metric has only two conditions: Red or Green. A Green value, of course, indicates no increased risk. A red value indicates the patient has between a 4 and 6.7-fold increase in risk during the next 5.1 years.

Table 5

Patient Name:
Gender: M
Date of Exam
Date of Birth: /1955
Referring Physician:

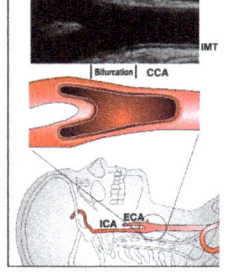

Patient Age	62	Patient IMT	0.79 mm
Arterial Age	64	Normal IMT	< .50 mm

CV Event Risk   All measurements in mm

Test Criteria:	Normal	Moderate	High	Last Visit*	Alert Value*
Early Event Risk[++]			2.8		2.5
Average CCA Mean IMT		0.79			0.73
Average CCA Max Region		0.89			0.75
Plaque Burden**			8.7		

Comments: The following values are the largest intima-media thickness (IMT) measurements found in each carotid artery segment. Any measurement equal to or 1.3mm is defined as 'plaque' and is characterized as being: S = Soft; H = Heterogeneous; or E = Echogenic (includes mineral deposits like calcium). All measurements are in millimeters.

Right CCA .8; Bulb 1.4 H; Internal Carotid 2.8 H
Left CCA .9; Bulb 2.5 H; Internal Carotid 2.0 H
Doppler was used bilaterally.

As shocking as this may be at face value, one must keep this metric in perspective. We often refer to this metric as the 'tie-breaker' metric. At its simplest level we can take it at face value. The metric is dynamic in that the alert value associated with it changes based upon each patient's chronological age and gender. The older the chronological age of the patient, the higher the correlated Alert Value and visa versa.

One way to think about this is by reducing to the ridiculous. An infant has zero or nearly zero risk of experiencing an atherosclerotic clinical event in the next five years. So, that infant's risk multiplied by 4 to 6.7 (times zero) . . . is still zero. By contrast, a 4 to 6.7-fold increase risk in a 60-year-old male with family history of disease poses a much different scenario. We may choose to treat this patient more aggressively.

This metric was developed by professor Damiano Baldassarre in his Italian Lipid clinic (Baldassarre, 2007). Dr. Baldassarre was attempting to marry CIMT measurements to the Framingham risk scores. After looking at data from patients who had experienced a clinical event, he mathematically developed a CIMT measurement for each decade of life and gender which he referred to as the "Best Threshold Value" (BTV). Patients with a Framingham risk score ≥ 10% and who exceeded this BTV, presented with an increased Hazard ratio of 6.7 or nearly a 7-fold increase in risk of clinical event in the next 5 years (± 2.3 years). Patients with either a Framingham risk score ≥ 10% OR a single CIMT measurement exceeding the BTB (or the Alert Value on the CardioRisk Scan Patient Results report) had an increase of at least a 4-fold hazard ratio. Patients who met both conditions (≥ 10% Framingham Risk Score AND exceeded the BTV) had nearly a 7-fold increase in risk of a clinical event in the next 5.1 years (± 2.3 years).

Once again, the metric provides an interesting tie-breaker when used in conjunction with the other values. In younger patients, it probably has limited utility, but in patients ≥ 45 years of age, or those with several or multiple other risk factors, this metric could provide a tie-breaker of sorts which could direct a more aggressive therapeutic treatment plan.

Table 6

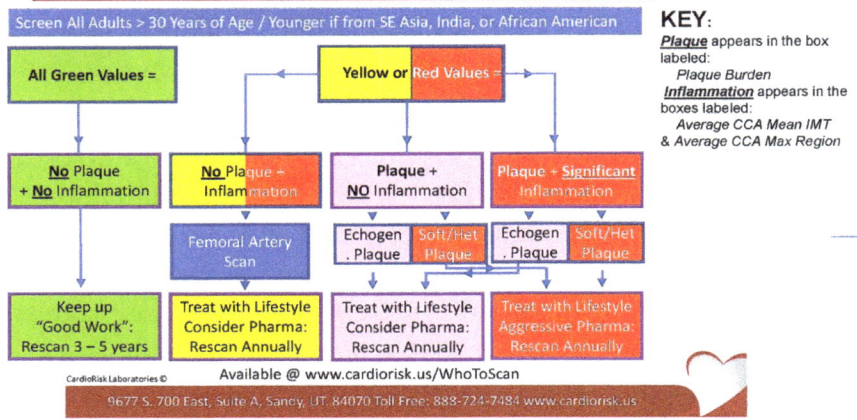

Taken together, the CardioRisk Scan Patient Results report provides much more data and more detailed data than does a standard CIMT exam. The test provided by Cardiorisk is accurate to 0.002mm as demonstrated in peer-reviewed, double-blind, performance-based certifications. Data from CardioRisk has been used in nearly a hundred different peer-reviewed journal articles and can be trusted as an important diagnostic and monitoring tool in both asymptomatic patients as well as those who present with more severe disease.

The first batch of patient results a clinician receives can be a daunting task. Absent the specific training above and below some of the results can be confusing and can appear to conflict with each other. For example, below are two scenarios which present data that, at first glance, may appear to conflict with each other. They are the most common questions we receive from physicians. Understanding the nuance outlined in these two scenarios is important to optimize the use of this data in your own practice.

Scenario 1: Plaque / No Inflammation.

Table 7

Date of Birth: /1940
Referring Physician:

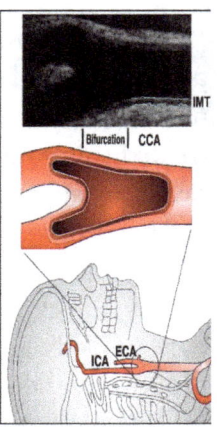

Patient Age	77	Patient IMT	0.68 mm
Arterial Age	53	Normal IMT	< 50 mm

Test Criteria:	Normal	Moderate	High	Last Visit	Alert Value*
Early Event Risk[++]	2.2				3
Average CCA Mean IMT	0.68				0.73
Average CCA Max Region	0.72				0.75
Plaque Burden**			5.2		

CV Event Risk   All measurements in mm

Comments: The following values are the largest intima-media thickness (IMT) measurements found in each carotid artery segment. Any measurement equal to or 1.3mm is defined as 'plaque' and is characterized as being: S = Soft; H = Heterogeneous; or E = Echogenic (includes mineral deposits like calcium). All measurements are in millimeters.

Right CCA .7; Bulb 1.4 E; Internal Carotid 1.1
Left CCA .7; Bulb 2.2 E; Internal Carotid 1.6 E
Doppler was used bilaterally.

When first looking at this patient's results and following the Therapeutic Recommendations Based on Results shown in Table 6, we should look at the patient's Plaque Burden score of 5.2, revealing that this patient has a large or significant amount of atherosclerotic plaque. A look at the inflammatory markers on the report (e.g. Average CCA Mean IMT, and Average CCA Max Region) show a male patient who has little if any inflammation. How is this possible? Given our understanding of the pathophysiology of this disease, how did this patient develop plaque absent a significant amount of inflammation?

The answer is . . . it is highly unlikely he did. At some point in time, this patient had to have a significant amount of inflammation prior to the formation of these plaques. The fact that there is no longer any inflammation infers that this patient has been managed effectively. It is likely this patient had a medical intervention (i.e. pharmacological and maybe even a significant lifestyle intervention) sometime in their past. The result of that intervention is that the plaques morphed from their initial soft and echolucent state, to being completely echogenic and hard. They are now healed plaques.

The inflammation which undoubtedly appeared throughout this patient's vasculature, has been arrested. This is evidence of a well-managed patient. We celebrate these patients and if you are the one who treated this patient, you should pat yourself on the back. It is likely you saved, or at the very least, you extended his life. Although the patient still has atherosclerosis (as evidenced by his plaque), he is no longer in an active or pro-disease state as his inflammation has been attenuated. This means that although we need to continue to monitor his atherosclerosis, it is unlikely he will develop new plaques as the underlying disease process that leads to plaque formation is in check. Clinically, the goal for this patient is to keep up the good work and to monitor his disease annually to assure that the inflammation doesn't begin to increase again.

Scenario 2: Inflammation / No Plaque.

Table 8

Patient Name:
Gender: F
Date of Exam
Date of Birth: /1963
Referring Physician:

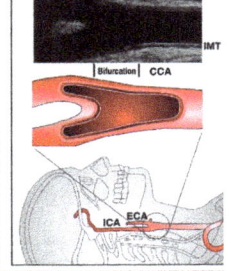

Patient Age	52	Patient IMT	0.90 mm
Arterial Age	>80	Normal IMT	< 50 mm

Test Criteria:	Normal	Moderate	High	Last Visit*	Alert Value*
	CV Event Risk			All measurements in mm	
Early Event Risk**	1.0				2.1
Average CCA Mean IMT			0.90		0.73
Average CCA Max Region			1.02		0.75
Plaque Burden**	NONE				

Comments: The following values are the largest intima-media thickness (IMT) measurements found in each carotid artery segment. Any measurement equal to or 1.3mm is defined as 'plaque' and is characterized as being: S = Soft; H = Heterogeneous; or E = Echogenic (includes mineral deposits like calcium). All measurements are in millimeters.

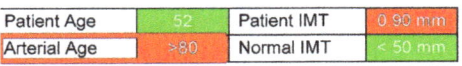

Right CCA .8; Bulb .9; Internal Carotid .7
Left CCA 1.0; Bulb .7; Internal Carotid 1.0
Doppler was used bilaterally.

When first looking at this patient's results and following the Therapeutic Recommendations Based on Results shown in Table 8, we should look at the patient's Plaque Burden score – and we can note that this patient has no identifiable plaque. A look at this patient's inflammatory markers on the report (e.g. *Average CCA Mean IMT, and Average CCA Max Region*) reveal a patient who has a large amount of inflammation. How is this possible? How can they have so much inflammation but no plaque?

This is a patient who is getting worse. Even absent a prior exam, we can tell this patient is progressing in the wrong direction. The amount of inflammation in this patient's report is evidence of active phagocytosis. They are in a pro-disease state. Absent an aggressive intervention, this disease has no choice but to continue its pathophysiologic disease pathway and eventually create multiple plaques. While we don't know from this report what is causing the inflammation in the wall of her arteries – we know that something must be responsible. At this point in time, it would be prudent to conduct an expanded list of blood bio monitors to ascertain the root cause of this inflammation. It would also be prudent to look at other vascular beds to see if she has plaque in her coronary arteries (Coronary Calcium Score) or in her femoral arteries (Femoral IMT scan). Additional cardiovascular testing is not necessarily indicated – but we absolutely need to get at the root cause of this problem.

This is where the Bale/Doneen Method excels. Their preceptorship: https://baledoneen.com/attend/about-preceptorship/ is the absolute best material I have come across as far as identifying Red Flags, and other root cause of disease . . . and perhaps more importantly, what to do about them. Although I have no financial ties to their program, I have been attending regularly for over 10 years. If you can't find the time to attend their 2-day preceptorship . . . at least take a look at their book: The Heart Attack Gene : (https://www.amazon.com/Beat-Heart-Attack-Gene-Bradley/dp/1118454294). It is a comprehensive tome on heart attack and stroke prevention and I highly recommend it. I consider them good friends – but I honestly have not found better data presented at any of the hundreds of medical conferences I've attended.

Final Thoughts On Interpretation of Results

Deciding on who and how aggressive to treat is an important part of any clinician's practice. Up until now, the who to treat has been limited to those patients who present with significantly abnormal cholesterol, blood pressure, or pre-diabetic conditions. Unfortunately, this approach misses more patients than it catches. The addition of CIMT to your clinical practice can help you to identify up to 98.6 of the asymptomatic patients who need therapy or intervention (Belcaro, 2001). Table 6 on page 170 above, provides an easy-to-use algorhythmic approach to image guided therapy using CIMT. We hope you will find it useful as you adopt and implement CIMT testing into your clinical practice.

FINANCES: THE $80k BOTTOM LINE

Virtually any discussion of finances or revenue brings discomfort to the physicians I know personally. One can nearly hear the sucking noises invoked by the clamping down of one's sphincter muscles at the mere mention of revenue, profit, or margins. Sorry for that graphic image . . . but honestly, there are very few things that create more consternation among my provider friends than the discussion of profit.

Don't get me wrong, everyone understands implicitly that health care providers must generate revenue and profit. We just don't like to talk about it with our 'out loud' voices. Think about it . . . maybe, but discuss it openly??? Never!.

Profit, of course, is what happens when and if there is money left after paying for all the operational expenses. Why then is it such a dirty little word? Why must it only be discussed in hushed tones and behind closed doors and even then, only amongst peers? Why are profit and revenue the subjects that cause such deep distress and consternation on the part of so many providers?

Mike and I go back a long way. He is a board-certified Family Physician who has been in practice for 20 years. Mike put it this way: "It's not that I'm embarrassed to make a living – I just have so many patients I see who appear to be indigent . . . or at the very least they are living paycheck to paycheck – I just don't want to appear insensitive to their situation". Can you identify with that comment?

Listen, let me try to help you with this one. To get where you are today, let's rehearse the typical pathway: First, you had to finish 4 – 5 years of an undergraduate program where you had to place near the top of your class (at least > 3.0GPA) while carrying a full load of very difficult classes which most students steered clear of (e.g. Chemistry,

Biology, Physiology, Physics, Human Behavior, Anatomy, etc). These are not your easiest classes.

Then, you had to take a very comprehensive exam to test your knowledge in a wide variety of subjects. Remember the MCAT? If you scored less than 490 you probably didn't get in.

THEN you went through four very invigorating but difficult years of medical school where you learned the foundations of medicine, clinical methods, layers of medicine. You probably studied molecules, cells, cancer, hosts and defenses. Then you probably studied metabolism, reproduction, circulation, respiration, regulation, the brain and behavior, the skin, muscles, bones, and joints. You probably had to work on a cadaver or two and you had to demonstrate a comprehensive knowledge not just of what, but where each of the systems, muscles, tendons, bones, and organs of the body were located on that cadaver.

By your third year of medical school most of you were doing rotations where you spent 6 – 12 weeks cycling through a variety of disciplines exposing you to the vast array of clinical application for the knowledge you acquired in your first two years of medical school.

Only after completing the four years of medical school and, based on how you did in those four years, you could apply to a specialty where you would invest another 3 – 5 years to become clinically proficient at diagnosing and treating diseases. Subsequent to the satisfactory completion of your residency program or programs, you submitted yourself to rigorous boards: a comprehensive set of tests which challenged your knowledge in the broad range of subjects covered in your chosen specialty.

You probably took on mountains of student loans in order to pay for the most basic physical needs while you participated in the privilege of learning. Your spouse and children rarely saw you as you devoted yourself to these studies and the rigorous schedule imposed on those matriculating through these programs.

In the years that followed the completion of this formal training, you have maintained at least a minimum of continuing medical education hours to keep you abreast of the latest trends and scientific updates pertaining to your specific field and your expanded list of medical interests.

You do remember all that, right? Can you remember well enough to once again feel some of the pain associated with those sacrifices? The rest of us stand in awe of you . . . or we should! I hope you can also remember the excitement you felt at each successful matriculation to the next phase of your learning and professional development.

Given all that, and we both know that this, the prior few paragraphs, grossly over simplify what represents a sacrifice so enormous that only the few . . . a small percentage of the population . . . could bring themselves to qualify and complete it, . . . why in the wide world then, would you EVER apologize or feel any amount of guilt or consternation at getting paid or making an honest wage for this expertise? If this bothers you at ANY level . . . you simply need to **GET OVER IT!!**

Why would you <u>ever</u> allow a patient, who occasionally see themselves as particularly adept in their google search prowess, get away with minimizing your life's work? Don't do it! **<u>PLEASE</u>** don't do it.

You have earned the right through years of hard work and delayed gratification, to earn a living. Not a meager income, but a good one. You have earned the right to have your wages reflect well over a decade of concerted effort to be able to perform the tasks that each and every one of your patients expects from you. THEY expect you to be right. THEY expect you to be the expert . . . even though they will sometimes challenge your knowledge. THEY count on you to enhance and preserve the quantity and the quality of their lives. YOU will do this, often without so much as a 'Thanks', . . . but for the love of God . . . you will collect your financial reward without embarrassment and without any guilt. You have earned it. You do deserve it . . . and YES – I DO feel strongly about it!

Having said that, this book does not ask you to gouge your patients. It does not ask you to 'nickel and dime' them to death (whatever THAT means). You will simply offer your patients lifesaving services (tests) at reasonable prices. You will need to explain the service and why the patient should have them completed. Occasionally, the patient will need to pay out of pocket for some or all of the services.

We must remember, however, that the standard of care (e.g. that which will be covered by 3rd party payers), that lowest standard to which patients will hold YOU accountable, that low standard which is responsible for one disease, a disease which is nearly entirely preventable, . . . One disease that is responsible for approximately 1/3 of ALL deaths in the US . . . THIS is the current 'standard' most of your patients will receive absent a change in YOUR behavior.

Optimal care, on the other hand, that care which significantly exceeds the lowest standard of care, requires a higher degree of effort. It requires that one do MORE than what is asked or expected. It is simply irrational for anyone to expect that optimal care will not also cost more! It will generally NOT be covered by third party payers, nor should it be.

This does not mean it will not be affordable. It only means that it may require a bit more sacrifice on the part of your patients. This trade-off of priorities is fair. It is equitable.

How many movies or dinners a year would most patients be willing to give up to make sure that the leading cause of death is not THEIR leading cause of death? What price do you think your patients would be willing to pay to preserve and enhance the quality and quantity of their lives?

Also, how badly do you want to continue to treat patients who do not put a premium on their own health? Premium is not only expressed in terms of dollars . . . it is a function of life choices as well. Patients who will not follow prescriptive advice are a poor risk for you and your practice. Why do you continue to allow them to be your patients if they refuse to make little sacrifices for their own health? These are the questions that must be asked.

In reality, these questions should probably be asked relating to every class of disease. However, as it relates to this book, you need to get comfortable with asking patients to seriously consider three changes to what they are doing in terms of risk assessment: 1) You will ask them to look at some additional blood bio monitors, 2) you will ask them check their vascular function, and 3) you will ask them to look at the structural wall of their arterial vessels. That's it. Three minor changes to the way you practice and to the list of services they may be accustomed to receiving. These three changes will make a mountain of difference and add significant value to the perception they have of the way you take care of them.

Patients will not need to take out a second mortgage or sell the family car to be able to afford these changes. In most cases, the initial out of pocket cost will be less than a single night's dinner each month. Are you worried patients would not be willing to spend that on their own health?

My Family Physician friend Mike (who parenthetically practices in a historically indigent area made up of many foreign nationals who work hourly jobs of manual labor and seasonal work) told me: "In our 20 year experience with these tests, I have never had a patient say they were unwilling or unable to pay for this care. It is difficult for some, but those that care about their health figure out a way to have them done every year."

So why do patients say 'no' to some of the prescriptive advice they are given by their providers? That is the subject of another book that I want to give to you free of charge:

COUPON

This coupon valid for one Complimentary Copy of the book:

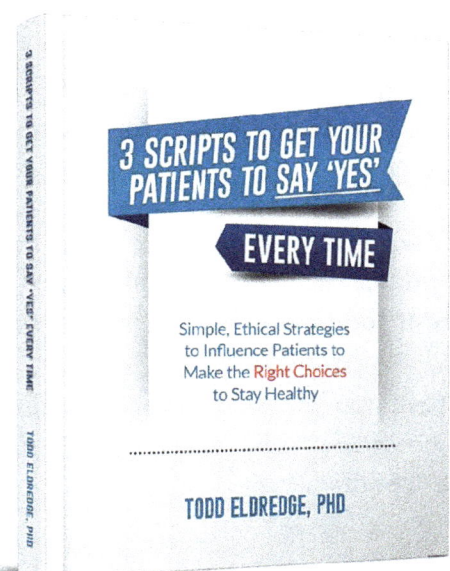

To Collect go to: CardioRisk.us/3scripts OR call CardioRisk 801-855-6775

I want you to have this because I know how much my friends struggle with this very issue. Please trust me when I tell you, and I say it with the utmost of respect, but . . . when your patients tell you 'No' it is **YOU** not them.

I'm not saying this to be hurtful. There are decades of research behind this. It is not the money, it is not the idea that you are suggesting. When your patients tell you 'No' it is because of how **YOU** are presenting the information and the specific word choices you make when you present an offer. This is classic human psychology.

The years of education you spent advancing your medical career was never meant to turn you into a sales person. The mere mention of that idea causes many to cringe and cower beneath the darkest covers.

Having said that, the skill of persuasion has never been limited to just sales professionals. The reality is that the gift of persuasion is perhaps the most important and underrated skill that can be acquired in any profession. It's just that sales people are so blatantly up front about selling and persuading that we tend to think of them as being unique in their persuasive skills.

Also - virtually everyone knows at least one obnoxious example of an over-bearing, hard-charging and offensive sales person. I would advance, for your consideration however, that those horrid examples of sales behavior are terrible examples of persuasion.

True persuasion, when done correctly, should feel a lot like asking your spouse to a movie. It should be natural, it should not feel coerced, the offer should be made with the foreknowledge that it is a good offer that will most likely benefit those involved in the decision, there is no manipulation, and there should never be any fear or anxiety associated with asking the question. The most important premise behind all correctly executed persuasive presentations is that they must be based on truth and conviction. When done correctly, persuasion will feel natural, non-contrived, non-manipulative because it's NOT and, most importantly, it will lead respondents to the most logical conclusion because it should always be in their best interest.

So once again, if your patients are telling you 'No', then **YOU** are the problem and I mean absolutely no offense by bringing this to your attention. We have to change the way we present information, and offers. If we are to be effective, we need to be careful in the choice of words we use because they DO make a difference.

In our practice management consulting we spend a great deal of time teaching staff (including or perhaps especially physicians and providers) how to present information. It makes a difference. It can make hundreds of thousands of dollars of difference every year. More importantly, if your prescriptive advice matters in terms of patient health outcomes . . . then it is crucial to their health!

We've already spent many of the prior chapters providing the rationale and clinical relevance pertaining to the offers you will make relating to cardiovascular disease. You will be asking your patients to change just 3 things. We are asking you to consider adding just two new tests to your toolbox. Hopefully you can see the advantage of making these changes.

Financially, you have earned the right to feed your bottom line, that line called profit is what you will show after you implement these changes. The numbers will show that making these changes and implementing them routinely into a testing and treatment algorithm of your practice of just 400 patients, will yield an annual profit exceeding $80,000.

I hope I have your full attention. This is not an exaggeration, these are the cold hard facts. I should add, that these are conservative estimates. Yes – it's true, by adding just two tests to your portfolio of routine exams on only 400 of your patients, your practice should experience an incremental annual profit exceeding $80,000. The reality is that it generates many times that amount in most of the practices we work with. It is important to note too that I am talking about profit, not revenue.

There is no mystery, no black box to purchase, no capital investment on your part to make this happen . . . just a modest change to your procedures to implement these tests into your practice. There will be a modest time investment for you to get your hands around how to use the test results to direct prescriptive behavior. We are not talking about weeks or months of your time . . . more like 15 – 30 minutes. We think the tradeoff will be well worth your time.

I hope you will take the challenge to learn how and why this is possible. I hope you will contact us immediately after reading this and ask us how.

You don't get these numbers by gouging your patients or by severely hampering their cash flow. If you do the math, we're only talking about $100 of profit for each test on each patient. This won't break most banks.

You are going to ask them to make a value exchange. In every case you will be asking them to give up a maximum of the equivalent of one dinner each month to cover the annual costs of these tests. I say a 'maximum', because they have to be prepared to pay for optimal care if their insurance company refuses to.   That is a small price to pay given the prospective trade off: being able to confidently enhance your ability to eliminate their risk of a future heart attack or stroke . . . especially when compared to their alternative (e.g. the lowest standard of care).

This approach moves each patient closer to optimal care, and the data suggests you can catch the vast majority of at-risk patients by implementing this three-step process.

There is absolutely no reason in the world you shouldn't be able to monetize and enhance your bottom line while you enhance your patient's care. You have earned that right – your education and years of preparation and delayed gratification should now be rewarded by the health care system and by the patients who count on you to provide them with optimal care. Own it!

CONCLUSION

The pernicious nature of this horrific disease cannot be understated. If we are not careful, we can become calloused and numb to the sweeping and wide-spread effects of its destructive tentacles. Heart Attacks and Strokes have unnecessarily but undeniably led the world in mortality, morbidity, and long-lasting sequelae for far too long. We must not allow ourselves to be complacent in the fight to unseat it from the list of leading causes of disease because IT is one disease that can relatively easily be defeated! Small changes can make a huge impact.

Never was this more clear to me than twenty something years ago when I learned to fly a plane. Shortly after completing my requirements for a private pilot's license, my wife and I, along with another couple left for Hawaii. It was my intention to rent a small aircraft from the Honolulu airport and take several tours of the islands including an inter-island flight.

Now most small planes didn't come with advanced navigation equipment. The most common navigational instrument was a VOR radio signal. The plane I rented in Oahu certainly did not have GPS navigation nor had iPhones, iPad's or the host of other personal electronic devices that assist pilots in their aeronautical pursuits today. Pilots simply learned to triangulate from several different VOR radio signals, and from this they could plot their navigational heading.

Inter-island navigation could be especially tricky because if you were off even a couple of degrees in your compass heading, you could miss the island entirely. For nearly 20 minutes of flight time between the island of Kauai and Oahu, I carefully and somewhat nervously watched for some sign of my intended destination on the horizon.

When your life depends on it . . . you learn to make the few minor course corrections quickly to avoid larger and potentially disastrous changes later because of not making the easier changes. Very slight changes were the only guarantee I had that we would eventually reach our intended destination.

So it is with Heart Attack and Stroke prevention. Small changes can make an enormous impact that will save lives. This book advocates small changes that you can make to your practice which will make a significant difference in the number of patients correctly identified as needing corrective action in the form of medical intervention. By catching more of your at-risk patient population, you will have the opportunity to treat more patients who, absent that treatment, would go on to experience cardio or cerebrovascular events. You will then have the capacity to monitor their progress to assure that the chosen intervention will amount to the positive health outcome both you and they desire. This will improve and renew the sense of satisfaction you have with the profession of medicine. Finally, it will improve the economics of your bottom line, a just reward for the sacrifices you made to gain the necessary knowledge to prevent these life altering events.

I hope you will find the courage to ask for help and let us assist in the implementation of these changes in your practice. We have helped thousands of providers just like you to do so. I promise it will be relatively easy and pain free – and you will not have to dip into your pockets for the 'privilege' of creating a new revenue stream. Adding these tests into your practice requires no capital expenditure, no purchase of equipment, it just takes a commitment to make a few minor changes.

I wish you the very best in your endeavor to save lives. I hold you in the utmost respect and admiration. I have a great sense of the many sacrifices you have made to get here, and I am genuinely interested in helping you to get more enjoyment out of your practice, and more financial benefit from your efforts. Mostly though, I am committed to your quest to eradicate this unnecessary disease from the world . . . beginning first with the patients in your practice.

May God bless you in your continued endeavors.

REFERENCES

Akosah, K. S. (2003). Preventing Myocardial Infarction in the Young Adult in the First Place: How Do the National Cholesterol Education Panel III Guidelines Perform? . JACC , Vol. 41, No. 9 May 7, 2003:1475-9. Doi:10.1.

Azen, S. e. (1996). Progression of coronary artery disease predicts clinical coronary events. Long-term follow-up from the Cholesterol-Lowering Atherosclerosis Study (CLAS). Circulation, 93:34 - 41.

Baldassarre, D. A. (2007). Measurement of carotid artery intima-media thickness in dyslipidemic patients increases the power of traditional risk factors to predict cardiovscular events. Atherosclerosis, 403-408.

Bale, B. D. (2016). High-risk periodontal pathogens contribute to the pathogenesis of atherosclerosis. Postgraduate Medical Journal, Vol93, Issue 1098. https://pmj.bmj.com/content/postgradmedj/93/1098/215.full.pdf.

Bastian, L. N. (1998). Diagnostic Efficiency of Home Pregnancy Test Kits. Archives of Family Medicine, 7:465-469.

Belcaro, G. e. (2001). Carotid and femoral ultrasound morphology screening and cardiovascular events in low risk subjects: a 10-year follow-up study (the CAFES-CAVE study). Atherosclerosis , 156(2):379-387.

Benn, M. N.-H. (2006). Improving Prediction of Ischemic Cardiovascular Disease in the General Population Using Apolipoprotein B. Arteriosclerosis. Thrombosis, and Vascular Biology. , 2006;27:661-670. https://doi.or.

Besler, C. D. (2014). Pharmacological Approaches to Improve Endothelial Repair Mechanisms. Expert Review of Cardiovascular Therapy, 6:8, 1071-1082, DOI:10.1586/14779072.6.8.1071. https://www.tandfonline.com/doi/abs/10.1586/14779072.6.8.1071.

Blankenhorn, D. J. (1987). The Cholesterol Lowering Atherosclerosis Study (CLAS): Design, Methods, and Baseline Results. Controlled Clinical Trials, Vol 8(4) 356-387.

Borhani, N. M. (1996). Final Outcome Results of the Multicetner Isradipine Diuretic Atherosclerosis Study (MIDAS): A Randomized Controlled Trial. JAMA, 276(10):785-791.

Bots, M. H. (1997). Common Carotid Intima-Media Thickness and Risk of Stroke and Myocardial Infarction: the Rotterdam Study. Circulation, 96:1432-1437.

Campbell, T. C. (2004). The China Study. Dallas, TX.: BenBella Books.

CDC. (2018). Centers for Disease Control and Preventon. https://www.cdc.gov/heartdisease/facts.htm, June.

Chambless, L. e. (1997). Association of Coronary Heart Disease Incidence with Carotid Arterial Wall Thickness and Major Risk Factors: The Atherosclerosis Risk in Communities (ARIC) Study, 1987 – 1993). . Am J Epidemiol . , Vol 146(6)483-494.

Chambless, L. e. (2000). Carotid Wall Thickness is Predictive of Incident Clinical Stroke. Am J. Epidemiol, Vol151(5)478-87.

Cheng, H. P. (2016). Effect of comprehensive cardiovascular disease risk management on longitudinal changes in carotid artery intima-media thickness in a community-based prevention clinic. Archives of Medical Science, 728-735.

Coskun, U. Y. (2009). Relationship Between Carotid Intima-Media Thickness and Coronary Angographic Findings: A Prospective Study. Cardiovascular Ultrasound, 7:59.

Costanzo, P. P.-F. (2010). Does Carotid Intima-Media Thickness Regression Predict Reduction of Cardiovascular Events? A Meta-Analysis of 41 Randomized Trials. JACC, Vol 56(24) 2006-20.

Crouse, J. R. (2007). Effect of Rosuvastatin on Progression of Carotid Intima-Media Thickness in Low-Risk Individuals with Subclinical Atherosclerosis: The METEOR Trial. JAMA, 297(12):1344-1353.

Danesh, J. C. (2018). Lipoprotein (a) and Coronary Heart Disease – Meta-Analysis of Prospective Studies. Circulation, 102:1082-1085. (https://www.ahajournals.org/doi/10.1161/circ.102.10.1082.

David, L. (2015). Gestalt Theory (von Ehrenfels), in Learning Theories. https://www.learning-theories.com/gestalt-theory-von-ehrenfels.html, 1.

DelPapa, N. C. (2008). Simvastatin Reduces Endothelial Activation and Damage But Is Partially Ineffective in Inducing Endothelial Repair in Systemic Sclerosis. The Journal of Rheumatology, 35 (7) 1323-1328. http://www.jrheum.or.

Dimmeler, S. ,. (2001). HMG-CoA Reductase Inhibitors (Statins) Increase Endothelial Progenitor Cells Via the PI 3-Kinase/Akt Pathway. J Clin Invest . , Vol 108(3):391-397 doi.org/10.1172/JCI13152. https://www.jci.org/articles/view/13152/pdf.

Eldredge, T. (2016). Data on file. A summary of over 50 peer-reviewed studies fully documenting these results will be provided to all those interested in the data.

Eldredge, T. (2018). Cardiovascular Wellness Management Success Plan: A Simple, 3-Step System to Diagnose, Treat, Monitor, and Eradicate Heart Attacks and Strokes While Growing Your Bottom Line. Sandy: Healthy Heart.

Espeland, M. O. (2005). Carotid Intimal-Media Thickness as a Surrogate for Cardiovascular Disease Events in Trials of HMG-CoA Reductase Inhibitors. Current Controlled Trials in Cardiovascular Medicine, Vol 6(3):1-6.

Falk, E. S. (1995). Coronary Plaque Disruption. Circulation, Vol 92, Issue 3 657- 661.

Fried, L. B. (1991). The Cardiovascular Health Study: Design and Rationale. Annals of Epidemiology, Vol 1(3) 263-276.

Furberg, C. A. (1994). Effect of Lovastatin on Early Carotid Atherosclerosis and Cardiovascular Events: ACAPS Research Group. Circulation, Vol 90(4)1679-87.

Giuseppe, M. G. (2001). Relation Between Blood Pressure Variability and Carotid Artery Damage in Hpertension: Baseline Data From the European Lacidipine Study on Atherosclerosis (ELSA). Journal of Hypertension, Vol 19(11)1982-1989.

Go, A. e. (2014). Heart disease and stroke statistics-2014: a report from the American Heart Association. . Circulation, 129(3), e28-e292.

Goldberger, Z. V. (2010). Are changes in Carotid Intima-Media Thickness Related to Risk of Nonfatal Myocardial Infarction? A Critical Review and Meta=Regression Analysis. American Heart Journal, Vol 160: 701-714.

Goncalves, L. e. (2012). Evidence supporting a key role of Lp-PLA2 generated lysophosphatidylcholine in human atherosclerotic plaque inflammation. Arterioscler Thromb Vasc Biol., 2012: 32: 1505-1512.

Greenland, P. A. (2000). AHA Conference Proceedings. Prevention Conference V. Beyone Secondary Prevention:Identifying the High-Risk Patient for Primary Prevention. Noninvasie Tests of Atherosclerotic Burden. Circulation, 101:111-116.

Grundy, S. B. (2001). NCEP Expert Panel on Detection, Evaluation, and Treatment of High Blood Cholesterol in Adults (ATP III) . https://www.nhlbi.nih.gov/files/docs/guidelines/atp3xsum.pdf, 1-25.

Heslop, C. F. (2010). Myeloperoxidase and C-reactive protein have combined utility for long-term prediction of cardiovascular mortality after coronary angiography. Journal of the American College of Cardiology. , 55 (11): 1102–9. do.

Honda, O. S. (2004). Echolucent Carotid Plaques Predict Future Coronary Events in Patients With Coronary Artery Disease. JACC, Vol 43(7)1177-84.

Johnsen, S. M. (2007). Carotid Atherosclerosis Is a Stronger Predictor of Myocardial Infarction in Women Than in Men. Stroke, Vol 38(11) 2873-2880.

Kastelein, J. S. (2005). Comparison of Ezetimibe Plus Simvastatin Versus Simvastain Monotherapy on Atherosclerosis Progression in Familial Hypercholesterolemia: Design and Rationale of the Ezetimibe and Simvastatin in Hypercholesterolemia Enhances Atherosclerosis Regression (ENHA. American Heart Journal, Vol 149(2)234-239.

Kramer, M. R. (2010). Relationship of Thrombus Healing to Underlying Plaque Morphology in Sudden Coronary Death. JACC, Vol 55(2): 122-32.

Landry, A. S. (2005). Quantification of carotid plaque volume measurements using 3D ultrasound imaging. . Ultrasound in Med & Biol , Vol 31(6)751-762.

Lauer, R. L. (1988). Factors Affecting the Relationship Between Childhood and Adult Cholesterol Levels: The Muscatine Study. Pediatrics, Vol 82(3).

Lorenz, M. B. (2010). Individual Progression of Carotid Intima Media Thickness As A Surrogate For Vascular Risk (PROG-IMT): Rationale and Design of A Meta-Analysis Project. American Heart Journal, Vol 159(5) 730-736.e2.

Lorenz, M. V. (2005). Carotid Intima-Media Thickening Indicates a Higher Vascular Risk Across a Wide Age Range. Stroke, Vol 37(1)87-92.

Mahon, M. T. (2017). New 11-Country Study: U.S. Health Care System Has Widest Gap Between People Higher an Lower Incomes. https://www.commonwealthfund.org/press-release/2017/new-11-country-study-us-health-care-system-has-widest-gap-between-people-higher, 1.

Mancia, G. F. (2013). 2013 ESH/ESC Guideines for the Management of Arterial Hypertension: The Task Force for the Management of Arterial Hypertension of the European Society of Hypertension (ESH) and of the ESC. Eur. Heart J., 34(2013) pp2159-2219.

Meuwese, M. d. (2009). ACAT Inhibition and Progression of Carotid Atherosclerosis in Patients with Familial Hypercholesterolemia: The CAPTIVATE Randomized Trial. JAMA, March 18 2009; Vol 301(11) 1131 - 1139.

Murphy, S. X. (2017). National Vital Statistics Report. Deaths Final Data. https://www.cdc.gov/nchs/data/nvsr/nvsr66/nvsr66_06.pdf, Vol 66, Number 6.

Naghavi, M. (2017). A review of State-of-the-Art in CVD Risk Assessment: Risk Factors vs. Structural vs. Functional Tests. Linked In, https://www.slideshare.net/Endothelix/why-should-we-measure-endothelial-function-76526309?

Naqvi, T. L. (2014). Carotid Intima-Media Thickness and Plaque in Cardiovascular Risk Assessment. JACC: Cardiovascular Imaging, Vol 7(10):1026-38.

Naruszewicz, M. L. (2008). Combination Therapy of Statin with Flavonoids Rich Extract From Chokeberry Fruits Enhanced Reduction in Cardiovascular Risk Markers in Patients After Myocardial Infarction. Atherosclerois , Vol 194;Issue 2:e179.

O'Leary, D. P. (1992). Distribution and Correlates of Sonographically Detected Carotid Artery Disease in the Cardiovascular Health Study. The CHS Collaborative Research Group. Stroke, Vol 23(12) 1752-1760.

Persson, J. F. (1994). Ultrasound as Determined Intima-Media Thickness and Atherosclerosis. Direct and Indirect Validation. . Arteriosclerosis and Thrombosis, 14: 261-264.

Peters, A. B. (2013). Carotid Intima-Media Thickness Studies: Study Design and Data Analysis. Journal of Stroke, Vol 15(1): 38-48.

Riches, N. A. (2010). Standardized Ultrasound Protocol, Trained Sonographers and Digital System for Carotid Atherosclerosis Screening. J of Cardio Vas Medicine, Vol 11(9):683-688.

Ridker, P. R. (2002). Comparison of C-Reactive Protein and Low-Density Lipoprotein cholesterol Levels In the Prediction Of First Cardiovascular Events. NEJM (2002) . . Nov 14, 2002., Vol.347(20):1557-65.

Ross, R. (1993). The pathogenesis of atherosclerosis: a perspective for the 1990s. Nature Publishing Group:, https://www.nature.com/articles/362801a0. http://dx.doi.org/10.1038/362801a0.

Ross, R. (1993). The pathogenesis of atherosclerosis: a perspective for the 1990s. Nature, 362:801-809.

Sachdeva, A. C. (2009). Lipid Levels in Patients Hospitalized with Coronary Artery Disease: An Analysisi of 136,905 Hospitalizations in Get With The Guidelines. American Heart Journal, Vol. 157(1)111-117.e2.

Sachdeva, A. C. (2009). Lipid Levels in Patients Hospitalized withCoronary Artery Disease: An analysis of 136,905 hospitalizations in Get With The Guidelines. AHJ - https://www.sciencedirect.com/scienc, Vol157, Issue 1:111-117.e2.

Sawyer, B. G. (2017). How Does the Qualtiy of the U.S. Healthcare System Compare To Other Countries? https://www.healthsystemtracker.org/chart-collection/quality-u-s-healthcare-system-compare-countries/#item-disease-burden-higher-u-s-comparable-countries-2, 1.

Smilde, T. W. (2001). Effect of Aggressive Versus Conventional Lipid Lowering on Atherosclerosis in Familial Hypercholesterolemia (ASAP): A prospective, Randomized, Double-Blind Trial. The Lancet, Vol 357(9256)577-81.

Smolders, B. L. (2007). Lipoprotein (a) and Stroke – A Meta-Analysis of Observational Studies. Stroke, 38:1959-1966. (31 Studies) https://doi.org/10.1161/STROKEAHA.106.480657.

Solutions, I. S. (2005). IntraMed Scientific Solutions.

Spence, J. E. (2002). Carotid Plaque Area: A Tool for Targeting and Evaluating Vascular Preventative Therapy. Stroke, Vol 33: 2916-2922.

Taylor, A. L. (2006). The effect of 24 months of combination statin and extended-release niacin on carotid intima-media thickness: ARBITER 3. Current Medical Research and Opinion, 2243-2250.

WHO. (2000). World Health Organizations Rankng of the World's Health Systems. http://thepatientfactor.com/canadian-health-care-information/world-health-organizations-ranking-of-the-worlds-health-systems/, Statistical Anex.

Zanchetti, A. B. (1998). Risk Factors Associated with Alterations in Carotid Intima-Media Thickness in Hypertension: Baseline Data From the European Lacidipine Study on Atherosclerosis. Journal of Hypertension, Vol 16(7) 949-961 JUL 1998.